European School of Oncology

Monographs

Series Editor: U. Veronesi

The European School of Oncology gratefully acknowledges sponsorship for the Task Force received from Fidia S.p.A., the discoverers and marketers of CRONASSIAL® (gangliosides), a drug experimentally proven to be effective in enhancing the intrinsic repair mechanisms of neural tissue in vincristine neuropathy.

J. Hildebrand (Ed.)

Management in Neuro-Oncology

With 7 Figures and 25 Tables

Springer-Verlag
Berlin Heidelberg New York
London Paris Tokyo
Hong Kong Barcelona
Budapest

Jerzy Hildebrand

Service de Neurologie
Hôpital Erasme
Université Libre de Bruxelles
Route de Lennik, 808
1070 Bruxelles, Belgium

ISBN-13:978-3-642-77880-3 e-ISBN-13:978-3-642-77878-0
DOI: 10.1007/978-3-642-77878-0

Library of Congress Cataloging-in-Publication Data
Management in neuro-oncology / J. Hildebrand (ed.)
(Monographs / European School of Oncology)
Includes bibliographical references and index.
ISBN-13:978-3-642-77880-3

1. Brain–Tumors. 2. Metastasis. I. Hildebrand, J. (Jerzy) II. Series: Monographs (European School of Oncology) [DNLM: 1. Nervous System Neoplasms–therapy. WL 358 M2652] RC280.B7M34 1992 616.99'481–dc20 DNLM/DLC for Library of Congress

Softcover reprint of the hardcover 1st edition 1992

Typesetting: Camera ready by editor

23/3145 - 5 4 3 2 1 0 - Printed on acid-free paper

Foreword

The European School of Oncology came into existence to respond to a need for information, education and training in the field of the diagnosis and treatment of cancer. There are two main reasons why such an initiative was considered necessary. Firstly, the teaching of oncology requires a rigorously multidisciplinary approach which is difficult for the Universities to put into practice since their system is mainly disciplinary orientated. Secondly, the rate of technological development that impinges on the diagnosis and treatment of cancer has been so rapid that it is not an easy task for medical faculties to adapt their curricula flexibly.

With its residential courses for organ pathologies and the seminars on new techniques (laser, monoclonal antibodies, imaging techniques etc.) or on the principal therapeutic controversies (conservative or mutilating surgery, primary or adjuvant chemotherapy, radiotherapy alone or integrated), it is the ambition of the European School of Oncology to fill a cultural and scientific gap and, thereby, create a bridge between the University and Industry and between these two and daily medical practice.

One of the more recent initiatives of ESO has been the institution of permanent study groups, also called task forces, where a limited number of leading experts are invited to meet once a year with the aim of defining the state of the art and possibly reaching a consensus on future developments in specific fields of oncology.

The ESO Monograph series was designed with the specific purpose of disseminating the results of these study group meetings, and providing concise and updated reviews of the topic discussed.

It was decided to keep the layout relatively simple, in order to restrict the costs and make the monographs available in the shortest possible time, thus overcoming a common problem in medical literature: that of the material being outdated even before publication.

Umberto Veronesi
Chairman Scientific Committee
European School of Oncology

Contents

Introduction

Jerzy Hildebrand

Service de Neurologie, Hôpital Erasme, Route de Lennik 808, 1070 Brussels, Belgium

Lesions of the nervous system are common in cancer patients; approximately 1 out of 5 patients with generalised neoplasia will develop a major neurological insult, most commonly caused by metastatic or toxic and metabolic disorders. The majority of these complications will occur in the advanced stages of the disease, when a definite cure is unlikely. Even in such patients, however, prompt management of the neurological disorders is important, for it may not only prolong survival but also improve quality of life.

Treatment of primary brain tumours is another important challenge in neuro-oncology. Brain tumours represent the second most common neoplasia in children and substantial progress has been made in the management of childhood brain tumours.

Management of cancer-related neurological complications is not only aimed at symptomatic lesions: it may also be prophylactic. The best known example of this is preventive treatment of lymphoblastic meningeal leukaemia. In other tumours, prevention of meningeal or cerebral metastases is controversial.

Also the management of symptomatic lesions is full of uncertainties and controversies. Many questions, such as selection for neurosurgery of patients with brain metastases, the place of laminectomy in epidural metastases, the best dose and schedule for intrathecal drug administration in the treatment of meningeal metastases, are still unanswered. Furthermore, in low-grade gliomas even the benefit of surgery and radiation therapy has not been convincingly demonstrated.

Therefore, although the aim of this mongraph is to report the state of the art of management in neuro-oncology, it must be stressed that many conclusive answers are still awaited.

In several neurological cancer lesions, early diagnosis is more crucial that the treatment modality. Early recognition of symptoms and signs leading to the discovery of neurological lesions is therefore an essential part of their management. This is a matter which is emphasised in several chapters of the monograph.

The quality of survival, especially in patients with neurological disorders, is also related to supportive care. Therefore, the benefits and unwanted effects of drugs such as glucocorticoids, anticonvulsants, anticoagulants or analgesics should be familiar to everyone who manages patients with cancerous neurological lesions. The monograph concludes with a chapter devoted to this subject.

As in the preparation of the previous European School of Oncology Monograph on Neurological Adverse Reactions to Anticancer Drugs, the editor was fortunate to work with an outstanding group of enthusiastic collaborators.

Treatment of Primary Brain Tumours

Jerzy Hildebrand

Service de Neurologie, Hôpital Erasme, Route de Lennik 808, 1070 Brussels, Belgium

The management of malignant primary brain tumours consists in a combination of surgery, radiation therapy and chemotherapy. The specific roles of each treatment modality will be reviewed by tumour type:

- Gliomas, including malignant and low-grade gliomas, oligodendrogliomas and ependymomas;
- Medulloblastomas;
- Primary brain lymphomas.

In assessing the efficacy of brain tumour therapy, especially chemotherapy, a distinction will be made between studies which evaluate the *rate* and *length* of tumour regressions (objective response), and those testing adjuvant treatments aiming to prolong *survival*, *free interval* (or time to progression, defined as the period from the first operation to the onset of progression) and/or the proportion of *long-term survivors*.

Phase II studies usually assess the rate and length of objective response and are performed in patients with recurrent tumours. Adjuvant therapy is tested in randomised phase III-type studies from the date of surgery.

Gliomas

Malignant Gliomas

In most trials, including the EORTC Brain Tumour Group studies, glioblastomas and anaplastic astrocytomas represent over 95% of cases, glioblastomas being about twice as common as anaplastic astrocytomas. The remaining 5% comprise, in our studies, gliosarcomas, oligodendroglioblastomas and mixed type malignant gliomas. Although it is recognised that these 2 tumour types differ in prognosis and probably in their response to treatment, they have been combined in most studies, and often cannot be analysed separately.

Surgery

Surgery not only establishes the pathological diagnosis, but also may prolong survival as well as improve its quality. All the large cooperative studies [1,2] have found that patients undergoing only biopsy have a shorter survival, but this may be due, at least in part, to patient selection. The EORTC Brain Tumour Group studies failed to demonstrate a difference in survival between patients who underwent "partial" or "total" tumour resection as based on the assessment of the neurosurgeon. However, the apparent benefit of a more radical tumour removal has been demonstrated in many trials [1,3,4] including a BTCG study where the residual tumour volume was assessed by post-operative CT-scans [5].

In patients with recurrent malignant gliomas a second operation is performed with increasing frequency. Encouraging results have been published by Harsh et al. [6] both in glioblastomas and anaplastic astrocytomas. However, these results have been obtained in a highly selected group of patients.

Radiation Therapy

The efficacy of radiation therapy, which has been used for decades as an adjuvant treat-

Table 1. Randomised trials testing radiation therapy in malignant gliomas

Scheduled treatment	No. pts.	Median survival	Ref.
Surgery alone	42	17 weeks	[8]
Surgery + 5000 to 6000 cGy	93	37.5 weeks*	
Surgery alone	17	5.4 months	[9]
Surgery + 5000 cGy	20	7.5 months*	
Surgery alone	38	6.1 months	[10]
Surgery + 4500 cGy	35	10.5 months*	
CCNU 130 mg/m^2/d every 8 weeks	22	6.6 months	[11]
CCNU + 5000 cGy	19	12.0 months*	
BCNU 80 mg/m^2 + vincristine 1.4 mg/m2 on days 1 and 8 every 5 to 8 weeks	16	30 weeks	[12]
BCNU + 6000 cGy	17	44.5 weeks	
CCNU 100 to 130 mg/m^2/d every 6 to 8 weeks	27	8.4 months	[13]
CCNU + 5000 cGy	26	11.9 months	

Only the arms comparing radiation therapy combined to surgery or chemotherapy and the corresponding controls have been selected in this table
* statistically significant at least at 0.05 level

ment in malignant gliomas, was demonstrated in a prospective randomised trial only in 1972 [7]. Since then, a doubling in survival time has been confirmed in studies comparing either surgery alone with surgery plus radiation therapy or chemotherapy with chemo- and radiation therapy. The results are summarised in Table 1. Even in trials where the level of statistical significance has not been reached, a marked trend in favour of radiation therapy was observed (Table 1). In addition, the BTCG studies have demonstrated a dose-response relationship up to 6000 cGy.

As radiation therapy is at the present the most effective adjuvant treatment in malignant gliomas, numerous attempts have been made to increase its efficacy. They include the use of radiosensitisers of anoxic cells [14-17], other potential radiosensitisers such as cisplatin [18], changes in fractionation [19], the administration of chemotherapy before irradiation [20] and the increase of total dose from 6000 to 7000 cGy [21]. However, despite all these efforts 6000 cGy delivered in 30 fractions in 6 weeks remains the standard therapy. Because of the growing concern raised by the increased number of observations of dementia attributed to post-operative irradiation and possibly due to combination with chemotherapy [22], and the fact that the vast majority of malignant gliomas recur locally [23], the size of irradiation fields has been reduced from whole-brain irradiation to the tumour bed plus a 2-3 cm security margin in most centres. The improved localisation of tumour by various neuro-imaging techniques, including the PET scan, have also contributed to the reduction of irradiation fields. Factors predicting the response of malignant gliomas to radiation therapy are largely unknown; however, at least 2 studies have indicated greater benefit in younger patients [24,25].

Interstitial Irradiation and Stereotactic Radio-Surgery

In malignant gliomas, external irradiation is usually given within a few weeks of surgery. Interstitial irradiation (or brachytherapy) using iodine-125 or iridium-192 implants has been, so far, primarily used in recurrent tumours. Encouraging results have been reported by Larson et al. [26] with a median survival after recurrence of 52 weeks for glioblastomas and 153 for anaplastic astrocytomas compared to 28 and 51 weeks, respectively, following chemotherapy alone of unmatched retrospective controls. Comparable results have been reported by Loefler et al. [27] with approximately half of the patients surviving at 18 months. Focal radionecrosis frequently follows this treatment and requires reoperation. A study comparing external irradiation with a combination of external plus interstitial irradiation after first operation is in progress [28]. Stereotactic radio-surgery either with or without linear accelerator is another form of focal radiation therapy delivered in a single high dose to a stereotactically localised intracranial volume. The number of conditions amenable to this treatment modality has increased [29]. Although the treatment still primarily adresses vascular malformations, functional disorders such as pain, or truly benign tumours, stereotactic radio-surgery has been used in malignant gliomas [30,31] either as a "boost" to conventional external radiation therapy [30] or in the treatment of recurrent tumours. This technique, however, is only applicable to small tumours and is at present not suitable for the majority of malignant gliomas.

Chemotherapy and Immunotherapy

Phase II trials

These studies, which assess the rate and the length of objective response, are usually performed in patients with recurrent tumours.

Single-agent chemotherapy

The results of studies using single-agent chemotherapy are summarised in Table 2.

Table 2. Systemic single-agent chemotherapy in recurrent malignant gliomas

Agent	Usual, scheduled doses (mg/m^2)	REMISSIONS %	length (mo)	Refs.
BCNU	80 to 130 x 3 q 6-8 weeks	47-60*	9	[32,33]
CCNU	120 to 130 q 6 weeks	19-44*	6-8	[33-37]
Methyl CCNU	130 to 170 q 6-8 weeks	50* (R=18%, S=32%)	8+	[38]
PCNU	90 to 100 q 6-8 weeks	69* (R=27%, S=42%)	6	39
HeCNU	130 q 5-6 weeks	55* (R=20%, S=32%)	9	[40]
Fotemustine	100 weekly x 3 then q 3 weeks	74* (R=26%, S=47%)	8	[41]
Procarbazine	150 to 200 daily for 21 days	0-52*	6-8	[33,37,42,43]
AZQ	10 to 40 weekly	6-52* (R=24%, S=28%)	5-9	[44-48]
Carboplatin	450 q 4 weeks	40 (R=10%, S=30%)	6	[49]
DDMP	75 weekly x 5	7	variable	[50]

* Tumour regressions plus stabilisations
R = regression rate; S = stabilisation rate; AZQ = diaziquone; DDMP = 2,4-diamino-5-3',4'-dichlorophenyl-6-methylpyrimidine

The differences between the studies mostly concern the rate rather than the length of objective responses. Although there are many potential reasons for these differences, the main one appears to be the criteria chosen in defining objective response. In some studies clinical responses correspond to regression or stabilisation of neurological signs and in others, including ours, only patients with a clear-cut clinical improvement persisting at least 4 weeks after corticosteroid discontinuation were considered as having achieved a response. The role of the definition chosen to define a remission is illustrated by a more recent study with HeCNU [40], where 30% of patients stabilised but only 20% improved. Similar proportions were previously reported for methyl-CCNU [38] and PCNU [39]. The use of brain CT-scan probably provides a more accurate evaluation of tumour volume variation, with a 50% decrease of the contrast-enhanced area being considered as partial response, while its total disappearance is required for complete response. In our previously mentioned study [40], complete radiological responses were observed only in patients whose neurological examination remained improved after a complete discontinuation of corticosteroids. Next to nitrosourea-derivatives which are the most effective agents, procarbazine is often considered as the second most active drug [33,43], although its activity has been recently reassessed [42]. In our own experience, and in the EORTC Brain Tumour Group studies, we have only observed stabilisations. No patient who failed on nitrosoureas showed an objective response to procarbazine [37]. The response rate obtained with AZQ varies widely [44-48], but this agent, as well as carboplatin [49], is clearly less active than nitrosoureas. The experience with DDMP, an antimetabolite which readily crosses the blood-brain barrier, is limited. This agent appears to have a weak but definite activity in malignant gliomas [50].

Combination chemotherapy

The heterogeneity of the malignant brain gliomas and the rapidly developing resistance to nitrosoureas are the best rationale for combining several antineoplastic drugs. Yet, despite promising results observed in non-randomised studies, prospective and controlled trials failed to unequivocally establish the superiority of various combinations over single nitrosoureas in malignant gliomas [51,52]. It is noteworthy that combinations of water-soluble drugs such as vincristine and cyclophosphamide [53] have been reported to be active in recurrent gliomas in childhood.

Autologous bone marrow transplantation

Bone marrow hardly ever contains neoplastic cells in patients with malignant gliomas. Thus, autologous bone marrow grafts may be performed to allow doses of anticancer drugs to overcome haematological toxicity. This procedure has been tested in several studies using CCNU [54], BCNU [55,56] or etoposide [57], and all have demonstrated the feasibility of this method. However, because of the relatively small size of these studies and the absence of control groups, the potential advantage of the procedure has not been established, and it remains uncertain whether larger doses of nitrosoureas mean greater efficacy.

Intra-arterial chemotherapy

It is assumed that drug concentration within a tumour may be increased by intra-arterial administration, and this has been demonstrated for a number of chemotherapeutic agents including BCNU, cisplatin and etoposide. The studies summarised in Table 3 were performed in patients with tumour recurrence and attempt to evaluate - clinically and/or by CT-scan - the rate and the duration of remissions. Comparison with results obtained when the drugs are given systemically is difficult, particulary as many patients treated intra-arterially failed to respond to previous chemotherapy [62-65] and the drug doses differ from one study to another. The overall impression is that even though the response rate following intra-arterial treatment may be higher, especially in trials where combination chemotherapy is used [66,67], the duration of the remission is not prolonged. Although systemic toxicity is lower, CNS toxicity consisting in focal encephalopathies and blindness due to damage to the ophtalmic artery is considerably higher [58,59,68]. In addition, the procedure is more difficult to re-

Table 3. Intra-arterial chemotherapy in recurrent malignant gliomas

Agent	Usual, scheduled doses (mg/m^2)	No. responders/Total ST	PR	CR	Response length (months)	Reference
BCNU	200 to 300 q 6-8 weeks	4/19	8/19	0/19	5	[58]
HeCNU	120 initial dose q 6-8 weeks	-	9/53	17/53	8.5	[59]
Cisplatin	100, twice monthly		7/9			[60]
Cisplatin	60 to 120 q 4 weeks	6/20	6/20*		4 & 8	[61]
Cisplatin	58-100 q 4 to 6 weeks	0/12	1/12	0/12	6	[62]
Cisplatin	60 (one course)	14/35	12/35	0/35	4	[63]
AZQ	10 to 20 q 4 weeks	4/20	2/20	0/20	3 & 8+	[64]
VP-16 (etoposide)	100 to 350 q 4 weeks	5/15	1/15	0/15	2 to 10	[65]
BCNU Cisplatin VM-26	≥ 100 60 175	1/19	13/19*		4	[66]
Cisplatin BCNU	150-200 once + system 300 CCNU		10/12*		4 to 19+	[67]

* partial plus complete responses
ST = stable disease; PR = partial response; CR = complete response

peat. This therapeutic modality remains, in our view, an investigational form of treatment for brain tumours, and appears most promising for agents with very mild neurotoxicity.

Immunotherapy

In 1973 2 prospective and randomised trials testing immunotherapy, one using saline tumour extract and Freund's adjuvant [9], the other irradiated autologous tumour cells [69], reported conflicting results. The essentially negative results of the largest trial [69] possibly account for a long-lasting decrease in interest for this treatment modality in brain gliomas. The current revival of immunotherapy in the treatment of malignant brain tumours is represented by the use of interferons, lymphokines, and lymphokine-activated killer (LAK) cells.

Interferons display, among other properties, growth inhibition and immunomodulatory activities. In human glioma cell cultures, interferon-beta appeared superior to interferon-alpha, and this form has been used in most clinical trials. Because of the lack of standardisation in doses, schedules, and routes of administration (intravenous versus intratumour), the activity of interferon-beta in malignant brain gliomas is difficult to assess quantitavely. The objective response rate, including stabilisations, may be estimated as up to 25%, but the mean duration does not exceed a few months [70-74]. Thus, the optimal use of interferon and its possible combination with other therapies, including chemotherapy, remain to be established.

Tumour regressions have also been reported after local administration of autologous LAK cells and interleukin-2 [75,76]. However, more recent clinical trials [77,78] failed to confirm these favourable results and have stressed the importance of both neurological and systemic toxicity. Systemic toxicity, however, has been overcome in the study by Hayes et al. [79] by the use of lower and repeated doses of interleukin-2.

Antibodies - especially monoclonal - have been used without much success, either alone or as targeting vehicles for radioactive or chemotherapeutic agents in the treatment of various tumours. The lack of tumour-specific antigens and the immunologic heterogeneity of tumour cells limit the efficacy of this approach. In brain neoplasias, the poor diffusion of antibodies in the tumour and the necessity to cross the blood-brain barrier to reach the cells deeply infiltrating the normal brain parenchyma constitute additional limiting factors. So far the most promising results have been observed in leptomeningeal carcinomatosis [80, see also the section on medulloblastomas]. A recent and interesting approach is the use of monoclonal antibodies directed against growth factors and/or their receptors, such as the epidermal growth factor receptor [81], which are abundantly produced by malignant astrocytes.

Adjuvant chemotherapy (phase III trials)

Adjuvant chemotherapy, added to surgery and radiation therapy, has been compared to control treatment consisting of surgery followed by 5000 to 6000 cGy radiation therapy in at least 15 prospective and randomised phase III studies. These data have been previously analysed [2,82] and the most encouraging results may be summarised as follows:

a) BCNU given to patients also treated by radiation therapy marginally increases the survival rate at 18 and 24 months by approximately 15% [8,83];
b) The median survival is moderately but significantly increased only by the combination of dibromodulcitol plus CCNU [84], admittedly in a relatively small number of patients.

A number of studies using either single agents [12,21,36,85,86] or combinations containing nitrosoureas [21,37,87-89] failed to prolong survival and/or time to recurrence and did not increase the percentage of survivors at 18 and 24 months. However, in malignant childhood gliomas, adjuvant chemotherapy consisting of CCNU and vincristine prolonged the median survival and statistically increased the rate of long-term survivors in at least one recent study [90].

Despite encouraging preliminary results, a randomised study performed by the BTCG demonstrated that intra-arterial treatment with BCNU was not superior to the systemic administration in terms of survival but was definitely more neurotoxic [91].

Several prognostic factors have emerged from phase III trials in patients with malignant gliomas. Three of them have been found consistently in virtually all studies analysed for this review. These are: age, performance or neurological status, and pathology. Younger patients, patients with a good performance status and those with anaplastic astrocytoma survive longer. At least these 3 prognostic factors should be reported in every therapeutic trial [1].

In conclusion, malignant gliomas should be treated by optimal surgical tumour removal followed by 6000 cGY radiation therapy given in 30 fractions to a localised volume. Adjuvant therapy tested so far is unlikely to prolong the median survival, but BCNU will increase the survival rate at 18 and 24 months by about 15%. Because the duration of the adjuvant chemotherapy has not been established and because of its potential toxicity, the author prefers to delay its administration until recurrence (unless patients are enrolled in a prospective trial). High intermittent doses of corticosteroids used during the free interval will not affect survival [92]. On recurrence, selected patients may benefit from a second operation, others from brachyradiotherapy. All may be treated with nitrosoureas, which will improve the clinical condition in about 20% and stabilise tumour progression in an additional 30% for 6 to 9 months. The advantage of combination chemotherapy or intracarotid chemotherapy over systemic administration of a single nitrosourea has not been shown for agents tested so far. Today, immunotherapy does not appear to be of practical use. Because the progress made in the treatment of malignant gliomas is so modest, one feels that these patients should be referred to centres with a special interest in this disease, where prospective trials aiming to improve their prognosis are performed.

Low-Grade Astrocytomas

There is no unanimously accepted definition for this group of tumours. In most studies they include well differentiated astrocytomas corresponding to grade II of the WHO classification. Pilocytic astrocytomas which have a particularly favourable post-operative outcome with 90% survival at 5 years [93] form a separate group of tumours. The lack of enhancement on CT-scan and the low uptake of fluoro-deoxyglucose on PET-scan [94] are

common characteristics of these tumours but do not reliably predict tumour grade in all cases [95,96]. Low-grade astrocytomas are characterised by an extreme variability in outcome and their optimal treatment is one of the most controversial issues in neuro-oncology [97].
Surgery is not curative, but some retrospective studies indicate that the extent of surgical removal is correlated with longer survival [98]. Tumour resection is justified in patients with increased intracranial pressure, neurological deficit due to mass effect, or seizures that cannot be controlled by medical treatment. However, in asymptomatic patients with indolent hemispheric gliomas diagnosed by stereotactic biopsy, the benefit of neurosurgery has not been proven. Equally controversial is the use of radiation therapy. Its effectiveness is based only on analyses of retrospective studies [99,100]. Such retrospective analyses have allowed the identification of poor-risk factors for 5-year survival and they include age over 50, male sex, biopsy alone, altered mental status and the absence of seizures [101]. The claim that radiation therapy can prevent or delay the transformation of low-grade into anaplastic lesions is purely speculative. Only prospective trials will determine the possible benefit of radiotherapy in low-grade gliomas and the appropriate doses. Two EORTC trials are currently comparing 2 doses of radiations, 5400 versus 4500 cGy, and early versus delayed radiation therapy with 5400 cGy.
In patients with signs of tumour progression or recurrence, there is probably more justification for surgery (often a second operation) or radiation therapy (if not previously given) when:

a) there is evidence of tumour progression;
b) the life expectancy is shorter and thus the risk of radiation-induced encephalopathy less relevant;
c) the recurrence may be an anaplastic transformation.

Interstitial radiation therapy has been advocated by Ostertag [102] but his large and encouraging experience is difficult to evaluate in the absence of a randomised control group.
Chemotherapy similar to that considered for malignant gliomas can be used at least in patients where the recurring tumours correspond to a malignant transformation. Reviewing the literature, J. Bloom concluded that low-grade gliomas were more sensitive to nitrosoureas than the malignant forms [103], and this was also our own impression [104].
In conclusion, the treatment of newly diagnosed low-grade gliomas is studded with uncertainties.

- Whereas symptomatic tumours should be operated, the benefit of surgery in indolent and asymptomatic lesions is uncertain.
- The benefit of radiation therapy delivered after the first operation or after stereotactic biopsy remains unproven.
- In patients with signs of tumour recurrence several therapeutic modalities are available.
- Tumour removal; often a second operation.
- External irradiation (if not previously administered) possibly combined with stereotactic brachytherapy.
- If the recurrence corresponds to a malignant transformation, chemotherapy similar in nature to that used in malignant gliomas.

Oligodendrogliomas and Ependymomas

These are 2 relatively rare gliomas, each accounting for less than 5% of all primary brain tumours. Whilst oligodendrogliomas are hemispheric and primarily frontal neoplasms of the middle-aged adult, ependymomas are predominantly seen in children and adolescents and originate most commonly in the fourth ventricle. In both tumour types pathological grading has been disappointing as a prognostic factor. Although the more aggressive forms are associated with nuclear polymorphism in oligodendroglioma, abundant mitotic figures and vascular proliferation and high cell density in ependymomas. However, younger age may outweigh pathology in oligodendrogliomas [105,106] and in ependymomas. Infants of 24 months or younger at diagnosis of an ependymoma have an extremely poor outcome [107].
The low incidence of these tumours and the poor reliability of prognostic criteria account for the lack of prospective phase III studies,

and for the difficulty of comparing phase II tirals.

Oligodendrogliomas

In a review of 323 cases, the overall median survival was 53 months [108]. This [108] and other retrospective analyses [105,106] indicate that surgery is the initial therapy in 80-100% of cases and that adjuvant radiation therapy (4000 to 5000 cGy) is given to more than 90% of patients [105,108]. Yet, the benefit of irradiation advocated by some authors [109] has been questioned [106].

At recurrence, retrospective analyses indicate that a second operation is common at least in lower grade forms [108]. More recently, the high sensitivity of the malignant forms of oligodendroglioma to a combination of procarbazine, CCNU and vincristine (PCV) has been reported; of 10 patients with recurrent tumour 2 had a complete and 8 a partial response [110].

Ependymomas

Despite the lack of prospective evaluations, surgery followed by radiation therapy (5000 to 5500 cGy) is the accepted therapeutic modality yielding 5-year survival in approximately 50%. The extreme figures recently reviewed by Lyons and Kelly range from 11 to 88% [111]. The prognostic importance of postoperative residual tumour, appreciated by imaging (not by neurosurgical reports) has been shown [107]. Cerebrospinal axis irradiation has been advocated because of meningeal tumour seedings but remains controversial. The incidence of leptomeningeal seeding varies greatly from one study to another; the average figure calculated for 385 cases collected by Bloom and Walsh [109] was 13%. High-grade ependymomas or tumours located in the posterior fossa are most likely to benefit from spinal irradiation.

In patients with tumour recurrence, partial and complete remissions of usually short duration have been obtained with chemotherapy, mainly cisplatin (Table 4).

In conclusion, extensive surgery should be performed in ependymomas and symptomatic oligodendrogliomas, but as in low-grade astrocytomas, its benefit in quiescent oligodendrogliomas has not been established.

In ependymomas, radiation therapy (5000 to 5500 cGy) delivered to the tumour site is an established treatment. The selection criteria for cranio-spinal irradiation remain controversial. In most centres, this treatment will be given to patients with undifferentiated ependymomas of the posterior fossa. In oligodendrogliomas, the role of adjuvant radiation therapy remains controversial. Chemotherapy is useful in patients with signs of tumour recurrence. In particular cisplatin has been demonstrated to be active in ependymomas, and the PCV combination in aggressive oligodendrogliomas.

Table 4. Cisplatin in recurrent ependymomas

Scheduled treatmen (mg/m2)	No. of patients (age)	Response ST	PR	CR	Length of response (months)	Reference
Cisplatin 60 on days 1 & 2 q 3 to 4 weeks	7 (3-17 yrs)	2	3	1	2-13	[112]
As above	15 (< 21 yrs)	4	-	3	3-15	[113]
As above	6 (1-3 yrs)	1	1	2	3-41	[114]

Medulloblastomas

Medulloblastomas represent about 20% of all intracranial neoplasms in children, but less than 5% of those in adults. They are treated similarly in children and adults. Medulloblastomas are characterised by a high proliferating fraction, which makes them sensitive to both radiation and chemotherapy.
Radical tumour resection is required whenever possible. Patients with residual neoplastic tissue have a higher percentage of recurrence [115,116]. However, it has not yet been proven conclusively that aggressive resection can annul the significance of larger tumour size at diagnosis [116]. Other factors defining the high-risk group are younger age (less than 3 years in the SIOP trial [117] and less than 4 in the CCSG study [116]), tumour size and its local and metastatic extension beyond the primary site at diagnosis.

Post-operative Treatment

Radiation therapy

Post-operative irradiation is the mainstay of the treatment of medulloblastomas. It is, indeed, the main factor which results in a 50-70% survival at 5 years and approximately 40% at 10 years. The standard doses are 5000 to 5500 cGy delivered in 30 fractions to the posterior fossa and 3500 to 4000 cGy to the rest of the cranio-spinal axis, with a possible additional boost to spinal deposits found during post-operative staging. In a recent French cooperative trial, the cerebral and spinal prophylaxis has been reduced to 2500 cGy [118]. However, a CCSG study had to be interrupted because of an unacceptably high number of early neuraxis failures observed in average-risk patients treated with 2400 cGy and no adjuvant chemotherapy [119].

Adjuvant chemotherapy

The results of 4 randomised and prospective trials are summarised in Table 5. In the two major studies [116,117] very similar radiation and chemotherapy schedules were used and these trials yielded comparable results. Both the overall and the disease-free survival at 5 years were not statistically prolonged when vincristine plus CCNU [117] or vincristine, CCNU plus prednisolone [116] were added to radiation therapy. In the SIOP study [117], however, the trend was clearly in favour of chemotherapy without quite reaching the level of statistical significance (p=0.07). In addition, in the SIOP and the CCSG studies adjuvant chemotherapy appeared beneficial in the high-risk group (Table 5). Similarly, the study of the German Pediatric Oncology Group [120] failed to show the benefit of 2 different chemotherapy regimens; the first given before and just after irradiation (sandwich technique), and the second as maintenance chemotherapy.
A fourth recently published study [121], in which radiation therapy was modified during the course of the study, used nitrogen mustard, vincristine, procarbazine and prednisolone (MOPP) as adjuvant chemotherapy. In this trial, MOPP administration marginally increased (p=0.07) the overall survival whereas the event-free survival was significantly increased (p=0.05) only in children older than 5 years. The benefit disappeared after 5-year follow-up, a trend also seen in the SIOP study.
Since the two largest cooperative trials [116,117] have been closed, high rates of remissions have been reported in phase II trials (which will be reviewed later) with drugs or drug combinations other than CCNU plus vincristine, possibly combined with prednisolone. Two studies, one using either cisplatin, CCNU and vincristine in poor-risk patients [122], or low-dose cyclophosphamide and vincristine [123] as maintenance adjuvant chemotherapy, reported very promising results. Unfortunately, these trials refer to historical controls. Finally, preoperative chemotherapy is used in infants and young children to delay radiation therapy.

Treatment of Recurrent Medulloblastomas

A number of phase II studies, some of which are summarised in Table 6, show that medulloblastomas respond to various agents and drug combinations. Although the results of these studies cannot be validly compared

Table 5. Adjuvant chemotherapy in medulloblastoma

Study arm	Scheduled treatments (mg/m2; unless specified otherwise)	No. of pts.	Survival at 5 years (%)	Disease-free survival at 5 years (%)	Subgroups who benefit from chemotherapy	Reference
RT	- 50-55 Gy* to post. fossa in 7-8 wks 35-45 Gy* to rest of brain 30-35 Gy* to spinal cord in 5-6 wks	145	53 (overall)	57	Partial (subtotal) surgery p = 0.007 Brain stem involvement p = 0.001	SIOP study [117]
RT + CT	- Same RT, CT: VCR 1.5 weekly during radiation, plus CCNU 100 on day 1 + VCR 1.5 on days 1.8 & 15 q 6 wks	141		41	Advanced (T3&T4) stages of disease p = 0.001	
RT	- RT similar to the SIOP study	118	65	50	More extensive tumours (T3 & T4) p = 0.006	CCSG study [116]
RT + CT	- Same RT, CT: VCR 1.5 weekly during radiations plus CCN 100 on day 1 + VCR 1.5 on days 1.8 & 15+ prednisone 40/day for 14 days q 6 wks	115	65	59		
RT	- 30-35 Gy to cerebrospinal axis plus 20 Gy to posterior fossa	43		59		GPO study [120]
RT + CT	- Same RT, CT: PCZ 100 on days 1 & 2 + VCR 1.5 on days 2 & 8 + MTX 500 mg on days 2 & 8	51		59		
RT + CT (maintenance)	- Same RT, maintenance CT: VCR 1.5 + CCNU 100 q for 7 months	15		59		
RT	- 54 Gy (48 Gy if < 3 yrs) to post. fossa - 35-40 Gy (25-35 Gy if < 3 yrs) to rest of brain - 30 Gy (25 Gy if < 3 yrs) to spinal cord	35		68	Children older than 5 yrs	POG study [121]
RT + CT	- Same RT, CT: - Nit. Must. 3 on day 1 8 q 4 weeks - VCR 1.4 - Prednisone 40 on days 1 to 10 - PCZ 50 mg on day 1 100 mg on day 2 100 mg on days 3 to 10 for 12 courses	36		57		

* Doses reduced by 5 to 10 Gy in children under 2 years. NS = not statistically significant; RT = radiation therapy; CT = chemotherapy; VCR = vincristine; PCZ = procarbazine; MTX = methotrexate; Nit. Must. = nitrogen mustard

Table 6. Chemotherapy in recurrent medulloblastomas

Agent	Scheduled doses (mg/m^2 unless specified otherwise)	Responders/Total ST	PR	CR	Length of remissions (months)	Reference
Cisplatin	60 on days 1, 2 q 3 to 4 weeks	1/11	1/11	2/11		[112]
Cisplatin	60 on days 1, 2 q 3 to 4 weeks	1/10	2/10	2/10	4.5 & 7.5 for CR	[113]
Cisplatin	120 q 4 weeks	3/14	5/14	5/14	8+ (median)	[124]
Melphalan	8 x 5 q 4 weeks			1/5*	14+	[125]
Cyclophosphamide	50-80/kg on days 1, 2 q 4 weeks			7/7*	6+ (mean)	[126]
Vincristine BCNU Methotrexate Dexamethasone	2-weekly x 5 100 (during maintenance) 500 (iv), 12 (it) weekly x 5 8/d x 36			5/5*	19-49	[127]
Procarbazine CCNU Vincristine	100 on days 1 to 14) 75 on day 1) q 4 weeks 1.4 on days 1, 8)			10/16*	10+ (median)	[128]
CCNU Cisplatin Vincristine	100 q 6 weeks 90 maximum 1.5 8 courses		2/6	4/6	18.5 (mean)	[129]
Eight drugs in one day			5/9	1/9	2-year progression-free survival: 24%	[130]

* partial plus complete responses
ST = stable; PR = partial response; CR = complete response

because the trials differ in terms of the patients' prognostic factors, they tend to show that remission duration is longer when combinations are used - a possible exception being the treatment with high-dose cyclophosphamide [126]. In addition to the studies where patients were treated with chemotherapy alone, remissions in recurring medulloblastomas were also observed in trials combining radio and chemotherapy [131]. An interesting new therapeutic modality consisting of 131^{I}-radiolabelled monoclonal antibodies (20 to 62 mCi) was used by Coakham and his group [80] in patients with recurrent medulloblastomas to treat meningeal spread of the disease. The effect of this immuno-radiation therapy is somewhat difficult to assess since it was combined with other treatments. Nevertheless, 5 of 12 evaluable patients responded with 2 complete remissions lasting 5 and 7 months.

In conclusion, newly diagnosed medulloblastomas should be treated with optimal tumour resection followed in children over 3 years by radiation therapy consisting of 5000 to 5500 cGy delivered to the posterior fossa and about 3500 cGy to the rest of the neuraxis. Lower radiation doses may be desirable, especially in younger children, in order to decrease the neurological toxicity of the treatment; however, they are probably less effective in controlling the disease.

In these chemosensitive tumours, chemotherapy is indicated:

a) in children under 3 years of age, to delay radiation therapy and thereby minimise its neurotoxicity;
b) as adjuvant treatment following surgery plus radiation therapy in high-risk groups;

c) in patients with recurrent tumours.

Both the optimum nature and length of administration of this chemotherapy remain to be determined. At present the author favours drug combinations of cisplatin, CCNU and vincristine or cyclophosphamide and vincristine. One must be aware that there is a price to pay for the high rate of cures achieved at 5 and 10 years, in terms of neuropsychological, endocrinological and growth disorders. The reported rates of cognitive disorders in treated children varies between 15 and 80% [132-134]. Differences in psychometric methodology and definition of criteria probably largely account for these variations.

Primary Brain Lymphomas

From the epidemiological and therapeutic point of view it is necessary to consider separately the CNS-primary non-Hodgkin's lymphomas (PNHL) found in apparently immunocompetent patients and those associated with immuno-deficiency conditions such as acquired immunodeficiency syndrome (AIDS), transplant recipients or congenital immunodeficiency states.

The CNS-PNHL are no longer a rarity, not only because the population of immunodepressed patients is expanding but also because in immunocompetent individuals the incidence of PNHL seems to have tripled during the last decade [135,136].

Immunocompetent Patients

Two recent reviews have addressed the issue of CNS-PNHL therapy [136,137]. Both emphasise 3 essential differences between the current treatment of CNS-PNHL and the therapy of brain tumours considered in the previous sections:

a) surgery is diagnostic and in many cases may be stereotactic biopsy;
b) currently the administration of chemotherapy precedes irradiation;
c) at least 50 percent of patients will respond to corticosteroids but unlike other tumours where steroids act on the peritumoural oedema, their effect in PNHL is cytotoxic. This cytolytic effect may occur within 24 hours, and although it is not sustained, may compromise the pathological diagnosis [138].

The lack of efficacy of surgical resection stressed by many authors [136,137,139-142] may be explained by several tumour features:

a) almost half of CNS-NHPL have metastasised when diagnosed. The most common secondary sites being the meninges or the ventricular space (found in at least one-third of patients [136,137]), and the posterior vitreous and retina (found in about one-fifth of cases [137]);
b) over 50% of tumours are multiple;
c) the majority of NHPL are deeply located in the periventricular white matter or basal ganglia, and are highly infiltrative.

Radiation therapy

The efficacy of radiation therapy has been shown since the mid-seventies [139,143], an era where chemotherapy was hardly used. Although the fields and the doses vary between studies and have changed with time, the results are fairly comparable and show that radiation therapy has moved the median survival from between 3 and 4 to between 12 and 24 months [137,139,142,144,145].

However, no cures were achieved even after irradiation with 4500 to 5000 cGy and the 5-year survival rate was less than 5% [146]. Considering the pathological similarity of primary cerebral and systemic non-Hodgkin's lymphomas, these results are surprising. Admittedly, the use of focal radiation therapy in patients with disseminated disease partially explains the results. Nevertheless, many relapses do occur locally in the brain [147], thus indicating that CNS and systemic non-Hodgkin's lymphomas respond differently to irradiation.

Regardless of treatment, survival has been correlated with:

a) pathological grade [135,140]: 80% of PNHL represent various forms of highly malignant types;
b) number [135] and size [144] of lesions, and the degree of tumour dissemination [147];
c) postoperative neurological and performance status [147];

d) younger age [137], but one has to keep in mind that, although CNS-PNHL affects all ages, its peak incidence occurs in the 6th and 7th decade [136].

The currently recommended radiotherapy consists of whole-brain irradiation with 4000 to 5000 cGy (e.g. 4500 cGy given over 5 weeks in 25 fractions [136,137]). A 1000 to 1500 cGy boost is delivered to the tumour bed if the patient fails to respond to prior therapy. Only if meningeal spread is documented (by CSF analysis, myelography or gadolinium contrasted MRI) may 3000 cGy be further delivered to the spinal axis. In addition, Hochberg et al. [137] recommend a 2000 cGy extension to the orbit if the vitreous or the retina are involved.

Chemotherapy

Pre-irradiation chemotherapy has been occasionally used to delay radiation therapy in infants and young children and to debulk voluminous chemosensitive tumours other than CNS-PHNL [148,149]; the latter, however, is the only tumour where it is systematically advocated in adults [136,137]. This therapeutic approach is based on theoretical considerations derived from treatment of non-CNS lymphomas, and therapeutic results obtained in PNHL of the brain.

The rationale for using high-dose systemic and intrathecal MTX derives from the experience gained in the treatment of metastatic lymphomatous leptomeningitis [152,153]. The dissociation in time of radiation and chemotherapy aims to decrease the risk of CNS-toxicity [152]. Two recent studies indicate the benefit of pre-irradiation high-dose MTX therapy.

De Angelis et al. reported 16 [153] and more recently 31 patients [136] treated with systemic MTX (1 g/m^2 on days 1 and 8) plus intrathecal MTX (12 mg total dose x 4 to 5, twice weekly). All patients received intrathecal MTX, regardless to CSF cytology. This chemotherapy regimen was followed by whole-brain irradiation with 4000 cGy. After the completion of radiation therapy, patients were treated with high-dose cytosine arabinoside (3 g/m^2). The median survival of 42 months compares favourably with historical controls, where radiation therapy was used alone. Gabbai et al. reported 13 [154] and more recently 22 [137] patients treated with high-dose MTX (3.5 g/m^2 every 1 to 3 weeks x 3) prior to radiation therapy. The median survival was superior to 27 months. In addition to MTX, whose activity was also shown in earlier studies [155-157], and cytosine arabinoside, several drugs and drug combinations are active in CNS-PNHL.

Table 7, which is not exhaustive, aims to illustrate the diversity of regimens and drugs

Table 7. Chemotherapy in primary CNS lymphomas

Reference	[136]	[137]	[142]			[158]	[159]	[144]			[160]	[161]
Regimen initials							CHOP				DEMOB	DHAP
No. of patients	31	22	1	1	1	5	8	7	2	3	1	4
Methotrexate	+	+									+	
Cytosine arabinoside	+											+
Vincristine				+	+	+	+	+			+	
Cyclophosphamide				+	+	+	+	+		+		
Doxorubicin					+	+	+	+		+		
Procarbazine or 6 MP										+		
Dexamethasone											+	+
Prednisolone				+	+	+	+	+		+		
ACNU									+			
BCNU			+								+	
CCNU												
Cisplatin												+
5-Fluorouracil									+			
Bleomycin				+								

+ = drug used; 6 MP = 6-mercaptopurine

which have been used with success in CNS-PNHL. It must be pointed out, however, that while these studies indicate that CNS-PNHLs are chemosensitive, their quantitative analysis must be tempered by the concomitant use of radiation therapy, the small number of patients studied and the fact that the frequently used CHOP regimen does not readily cross the blood-brain barrier and is known to lead to a high incidence of leptomeningeal recurrences [158]. Therefore, the optimal choice, sequence and combination of chemotherapeutic agents in CNS-PNHL has yet to be determined [136].

Immunocompromised Patients

The treatment of CNS-PNHL in immunocompromised individuals is similar to that considered for those with apparently normal immune defences, except for AIDS patients. The latter are statistically younger, have a lower performance status, and a shorter median survival [162]. Because about 90% of AIDS-associated brain lymphomas will respond to radiation therapy and patients will eventually die from other manifestations of the disease, chemotherapy is not commonly used in this group, and corticosteroids are restricted to the irradiation period.

In conclusion, when primary lymphoma of the CNS is suspected the administration of corticosteroids should be delayed until the diagnosis is made by open surgery or preferably by stereotactic biopsy. The diagnostic procedure is currently followed by at least 2 courses of intravenous MTX (1 to 3 g/m^2), and intrathecal MTX (12 mg total dose twice a week) should be given to patients with evidence of persisting leptomeningeal seedings. Chemotherapy is followed by brain irradiation with approximately 4500 cGy given in 5 weeks, and a 1000 to 1500 cGy boost is delivered if the response is not complete. Irradiation fields are extended to the orbit (2000 cGY) and/or to the spinal axis (3000 cGy) if metastases are found in these locations. It is quite possible, however, that spinal irradiation may be replaced by intrathecal chemotherapy alone.

The best sequence and composition of pre-irradiation and possibly post-irradiation (adjuvant) chemotherapy has yet to be determined. Recurrent tumours will respond to several drugs and combinations including regimens such as CHOP, which do not readily cross the blood-brain barrier. Whereas similar therapeutic recommendations will apply to PNHL found in immunocompromised patients, most AIDS-associated lymphomas are treated with radiation therapy alone together with corticosteroids given during the irradiation period.

REFERENCES

1 Byar DP, Green SB and Strike TA: Prognostic factors for malignant glioma. In Walker MD (ed) Oncology of the Nervous System. Martinus Nyhoff, Boston 1983 pp 379-395

2 Hildebrand J and Delecluse F: Malignant glioma in randomized trials in Cancer. In: Slavin ML and Staquet MJ (eds) Randomized Trials in Cancer. A critical Review by Sites. Raven Press, New York 1986 pp 583-604

3 Ammirati M, Vick N, Liao YL et al: Effect of the extent of surgical resection on survival and quality of life in patients with supratentorial glioblastomas and anaplastic astrocytomas. Neurosurgery 1987 (21):201-206

4 Vecht CJ, Avezaat CJ, van Putten WLJ et al: The influence of the extent of surgery on the neurological function and survival in malignant glioma. A retrospective analysis in 243 patients. J Neurol Neurosurg Psychiatry 1990 (53):466-471

5 Wood JR, Green SB and Shapiro WR: The prognostic importance of tumour size in malginant gliomas: A computed tumographic scan study by the Brain Tumor Cooperative Group. J Clin Oncol 1988 (6):338-343

6 Harsh GR IV, Levin VA, Gutin PH et al: Reoperation for recurrent glioblastoma and anaplastic astrocytoma. Neurosurgery 1987 (21):615-621

7 Walker MD and Gehan EA: An evaluation of 1-3-bis (2-chloroethyl)-1-nitrosourea (BCNU) and irradiation alone and in combination for the treatment of malignant glioma. Proc Am Assoc Cancer Res 1972 (13):67

8 Walker MD, Green SB, Byar DP et al: Randomized comparisons of radiotherapy and nitrosoureas for the treatment of malignant glioma after surgery. N Engl J Med 1980 (303):1323-1329

9 Trouillas P: Immunologie et immunothérapie des tumeurs cérébrales. Etat Actuel Rev Neurol (Paris) 1973 (128):23-38

10 Kristiansen K, Hagen S, Kollevodt T et al: Combined modality therapy of operated astrocytomas grade III and IV - confirmation of the value of postoperative irradiation and lack of potentiation of bleomycin on survival time: A prospective multicente trial of the Scandinavian Glioblastoma Study Group. Cancer 1981 (47):649-652

11 Reagan TJ, Bisel HF, Childs DS Jr et al: Controlled study of CCNU and radiation therapy in malignant astrocytoma. J Neurosurg 1976 (44):186-190

12 Cianfriglia F, Pompili A, Riccio A, Grassi A: CCNU-chemotherapy of supratentorial hemispheric glioblastoma multiforme. Cancer 1980 (45):1284-1299

13 Shapiro WR and Young DF: Treatment of malignant glioma. Arch Neurol 1976 (33):494-500

14 Bleehen NM, Wiltshire CR, Plowman PN: Randomized study of misonidazole and radiotherapy for grade III and IV cerebral astrocytoma. Br J Cancer 1981 (43):436-442

15 EORTC Brain Tumour Group: Misonidazole in radiotherapy of supratentorial malignant gliomas in adult patients: A randomized double-blind study. Eur J Cancer Clin Oncol 1983 (19):39-42

16 Hatlevoll R, Lindegaard KF, Hagen S et al: Combined modality treatment of operated astrocytomas grade 3 and 4: a prospective and randomized study of misonidazole and radiotherapy with two different radiation schedules and subsequent CCNU chemotherapy. Stage II of a prospective multicenter trial of the Scandinavian Glioblastoma Study Group. Cancer 1985 (56):41-47

17 Wasserman TH, Stetz J, Phillips TL: Radiation Therapy Oncology Group clinical trials with misonidazole. Cancer 1981 (47):2382-2390

18 EORTC Brain Tumour Group: Cisplatin does not enhance the effect of radiation therapy in malignant gliomas. Eur J Cancer 1991 (27):568-571

19 Shin KH, Muller PJ and Geggie PHS: Superfractionation radiationtherapy in the treatment of malignant astrocytoma. Cancer 1983 (52):2040-2043

20 EORTC Brain Tumour Group: Randomized comparison of radiotherapy versus VM-26 plus CCNU followed by radiotherapy in the treatment of supratentorial malignant brain gliomas in adult patients. Abstracts 15th International Congress of Chemotherapy, Istanbul 1987

21 Chang CH, Horton J, Schoenfeld D et al: Comparison of postoperative radiotherapy and combined postoperative radiotherapy and chemotherapy in the multidisciplinary management of malignant gliomas. Cancer 1983 (52):997-1007

22 Imperato JP, Paleologos NA and Vick NA: Effect of treatment on long-term survivors with malignant astrocytomas. Ann Neurol 1990 (28):818-822

23 Hochberg FH and Pruitt A: Assumptions in the radiotherapy of glioblastoma. Neurology 1980 (30):907-911

24 Sandberg-Wollheim M, Malström P, Stromblad LG et al: A randomized study of chemotherapy with procarbazine, vincristine and lomustine with radiation therapy for astrocytoma grades 3 and/or 4. Cancer 1991 (68):22-29

25 MRC Brain Tumour Working Party: Prognostic factors for high grade malignant glioma: Development of a prognostic index. J Neuro Oncol 1990 (9):47-55

26 Larson DA, Gutin PH, Leibel SA et al: Stereotaxic irradiation of brain tumours. Cancer 1990 (65):792-799

27 Loeffler JS, Alexander E III, Hochberg FH et al: Clinical patterns of failure following stereotactic interstitial irradiation for malignant gliomas. Int J Radiat Oncol Biol Phys 1990 (19):1455-1462

28 Shapiro WR, Green SB, Burger PC et al: Neuro-oncology. In: Paoletti P et al (eds) Recent Clinical Results in the Chemotherapy of Brain Tumors: BTCT Studies. Kluwer Academic Publishers, Dordrecht - Boston - London 1991 pp 147-152

29 Leksell DG: Stereotactic radiosurgery: Present status and future trends. Neurol Res 1987 (9):58-68

30 Lunsford LD, Flickinger J and Coffey RJ: Stereotactic gamma knife radiosurgery: Initial

north American experience in 207 patients. Arch Neurol 1990 (47):169-175
31 Rozental JM, Levine RL, Mehta MP et al: Early changes in tumour metabolism after treatment: The effects of stereotactic radiotherapy. Int J Radiat Oncol Biol Phys 1991 (20):1053-1060
32 Walker M, Hurwitz B: BCNU (1,3-bis(2-chloroethyl)-1-nitrosourea (NSC-409962) in the treatment of malignant brain tumours. A preliminary report. Cancer Chemother Rep 1970 (54):263-271
33 Wilson C, Gutin P, Boldrey E et al: Single agent chemotherapy of brain tumours. Arch Neurol 1976 (33):739-744
34 Fewer D, Wilson CB, Boldrey EB and Enot J: Phase II study of CCNU in the treatment of brain tumours. Cancer Chemother Rep 1972 (44):186-190
35 Reagan T, Bisel H, Childs D Jr et al: Controlled study of CCNU and radiation therapy in malignant astrocytoma. J Neurosurg 1976 (44):186-190
36 EORTC Brain Tumour Group: Effect of CCNU on survival rate of objective remission and duration of free interval in patients with malignant brain glioma. Final evaluation. Eur J Cancer 1978 (14):851-885
37 EORTC Brain Tumour Group: Evaluatin of CCNU, VM-26 plus CCNU and procarbazine in supratentorial brain gliomas. J Neurosurg 1981 (55):27-31
38 Levine M, Walker M, Weiss H: Intravenous methyl-CCNU in the treatment of malignant gliomas (phase II). ASCO Proc 1974 (15):167
39 Levin VA, Resser KJ, McGrath L et al: PCNU treatment for recurrent gliomas. Cancer Treat Rep 1984 (68):969-973
40 Georges P, Przedborski S, Brochi J et al: Effect of HeCNU in malignant supratentorial gliomas - a phase II study. J Neuro Oncol 1988 (6):211-219
41 Frenay M, Giroux B, Khoury S et al: Phase II study of fotemustine in recurrent supratentorial malignant gliomas. Eur J Cancer 1991 (27):852-856
42 Rodriguez LA, Prados M, Silver P and Levin VA: Reevaluation of procarbazine for treatment of recurrent malignant central nervous system tumours. Cancer 1989 (64): 2420-2423
43 Newton HB, Junck L, Bromberg J et al: Procarbazine chemotherapy in the treatment of recurrent malignant astrocytomas after radiation and nitrosourea failure. Neurology 1990 (40):1743-1746
44 EORTC Brain Tumour Group: Effect of AZQ (1,4-cyclohexadiene-1,4-diacarbonic acid, 2,5-bis (1-aziridinyl-3,6-dioxo-diethylester) in recurring supratentorial malignant brain gliomas. A phase II study. Eur J Cancer Clin Oncol 1985 (21):143-146
45 Taylor SA, McCracken JD, Eyre HH et al: Phase II study of aziridinylbenzoquinone (AZQ) in patients with central nervous system malignancies: A Southwest Oncology Group study. J Neuro Oncol 1985 (3):131-135
46 Decker DA, Al Sarraf M, Kresge C et al: Phase II study of aziridinylbenzoquinone (AZQ, NSC-182986) in the treatment of malignant gliomas recurrent after radiation. J Neuro Oncol 1985 (3):19-21
47 Eagon RT, DiNapoli RP, Cascino TL et al: Comprehensive phase II evaluation of aziridinylbenzoquinone (AZQ, diaziquone) in recurrent human primary brain tumours. J Neuro Oncol 1987 (5):309-314
48 Feun L, Yung W, Leavens M et al: A phase II trial of 2,5,diaziridyl 3,6-bis-(carboethoxy-amino) 1,4-benzoquinone (AZQ, NSC 182-986). J Neuro Oncol 1984 (2):13-18
49 Poisson M, Pereon Y, Chiras J and Delattre JY: Treatment of recurrent malignant supratentorial gliomas with carbodopa. J Neuro Oncol 1991 (10):139-144
50 EORTC Brain Tumour Group: Effect of DDMP (2,4-Diamino-5-3',-4'dichlorophenyl-6-methylpyrimidine) on brain gliomas. A phase II study. Eur J Cancer 1980 (12):41-45
51 Levin VA, Wara WM, Davis RL et al: Northern California Oncology Group Protocol 6G91: Response to treatment with radiation therapy and seven-drug chemotherapy in patients with glioblastoma multiforme. Cancer Treat Rep 1986 (70):739-743
52 Shapiro WR, Green SB, Burger PC et al: Randomized trial of three chemotherapy regimens and two radiotherapy regimens in postoperative treatment of malignant glioma. J Neurosurg 1989 (71):1-9
53 Longee DC, Friedman HS, Albright RE et al: Treatment of patients with recurrent glioma with cyclophosphamide and vincristine. J Neurosurg 1990 (72):583-588
54 Hildebrand J, Badjou R, Collard-Ronge A et al: Treatment of brain gliomas with high doses of CCNU and autologous marrow transplantation. Biomed 1980 (32):71-75
55 Hochberg FH, Parker LM, Takvorian T et al: High-dose BCNU with autologous bone marrow rescue for recurrent gliobastoma multiforme. J Neurosurg 1981 (54):455-460
56 Phillips GL, Wolff SN, Fay JW et al: Intensive 1,3,-bis (2-chloroethyl)-1-nitrosourea (BCNU) monochemotherapy and autologous marrow transplantation for malignant glioma. J Clin Oncol 1986 (4):6391 : a Southwest Oncology Group study. J Neurol Oncol 1985 (3):131-135
57 Giannone L and Wolff SN: Phase II treatment of central nervous system glioma with high-dose etoposide and autologous bone marrow transplantation. Cancer Treat Rep 1987 (71):759-761
58 Greenberg HS, Ensminger WD, Chandler WF et al: Intra-arterial BCNU chemotherapy for treatment of malignant gliomas of the central nervous system. J Neurosurg 1984 (61):423-429
59 Poisson M, Chiras J, Fauchon F et al: Treatment of malignant recurrent glioma by intra-arterial, infra-ophtalmic infusion of HECNU 1-(2-chloroethyl)-1-nitroso-3-(2-hydroxyl-ethyl) urea. A phase II study. J Neuro Oncol 1990 (8):255-262
60 Lehane DE, Bryan RN, Horowitz B et al: Intra-arterial cis-platinum chemotherapy for patients with primary and metastatic brain tumours. Cancer Drug Delivery 1983 (1):69-77
61 Feun LG, Wallace S, Stewart DJ et al: Intracarotid infusion of cis-diamminedichloroplatinum in the

treatment of recurrent brain tumours. Cancer 1984 (54):794-799
62 Newton HB, Page MA, Junck L and Greenberg HS: Intra-arterial cisplatin for treatment of malignant gliomas. J Neuro Oncol 1989 (7):39-45
63 Mahaley MS Jr, Hipp SW, Dropcho EJ et al: Intracarotid cisplatin chemotherapy for recurrent gliomas. J Neurosurgery 1989 (70):371-378
64 Greenberg SH, Ensminger WD, Layton PB et al: Phase I-II evaluation of intra-arterial diaziquone for recurrent malignant astrocytomas. Cancer Treat Rep 1986 (70):353-357
65 Feun LG, Lee YY, Yung A et al: Intracarotid VP-16 in malignant brain tumours. J Neuro Oncol 1987 (4):397-401
66 Stewart DJ, Grahovac Z, Benoit B et al: Intracarotid chemotherapy with combination of 1,3-bis (2-chloroethyl)-1-nitrosourea (BCNU), cis-diaminedichloroplatinum (cisplatin), and 4'-0-demethyl-1-0-(4,6-0-2-thenyliodeme-B-D-glucopyranosyl) epipodo-phyllotoxin (VM-26) in the treatment of primary and metastatic brain tumours. Neurosurgery 1984 (15):828-833
67 Kapp JP and Vance RB: Supraophtalmic carotid infusion for recurrent glioma. J Neuro Oncol 1985 (3):5-11
68 Mahaley MS, Whaley RA, Blue M and Bertsch L: Central neurotoxicity following intracarotid BCNU chemotherapy for malignant gliomas. J Neuro Oncol 1986 (3):297-314
69 Bloom HJG, Peckham MJ, Richardson AE et al: Glioblastoma multiforme: A controlled trial to assess the value of specific active immunotherapy in patients treated by radical surgery and radiotherapy. Br J. Cancer 1973 (27):253-267
70 Nakagawa Y, Hirakawa K, Ueda S et al: Local administration of interferon for malignant brain tumours. Cancer Treat Rep 1983 (67):833-835
71 Nagai M, Arai T: Clinical effects of interferon in malignant brain tumours. Neurosurg Rev 1984 (7):55-64
72 Yung WKA, Castellanos AM, Van Tessel P et al: A pilot study of recombinant interferon (IFN-B ser) in patients with recurrent glioma. J Neuro Oncol 1990 (9):29-34
73 Fetell MR, Housepian EM, Oster MW et al: Intratumour administration of beta-Interferon in recurrent malignant gliomas. Cancer 1990 (65):78-83
74 Mahaley MS Jr, Dropcho EJ, Bertsch L et al: Systemic beta-interferon therapy for recurrent gliomas: a brief report. J Neurosurg 1989 (71):639-641
75 Yoshida S, Tanaka R, Takai N and Ono K: Local administration of autologous lymphokine-activated killer cells and recombinant Interleukin 2 to patients with malignant brain tumours. Cancer Res 1988 (48):5011-5016
76 Merchant RE, Grant AJ, Merchant LH, Young HF: Adoptive immunotherapy for recurrent glioblastoma multiforme using lymphokine activated killer cells and recombinant interleukin-2. Cancer 1988; 62:665-671
77 Barba D, Saris SC, Holder C et al: Intratumoural LAK cell and interleukin-2-therapy of human gliomas. J Neurosurg 1989 (70):175-182
78 Blancher A, Roubinet F, Granchera AS et al: Immunotherapy adoptive locale dans le cadre des glioblastomas. Abstr. Réunion Internationale de la Société Française de Neurologie. Paris 13-14 juin 1991, p 22
79 Hayes RL, Koslow M, Hiesger EM et al: Biologic response to intracranial interleukin-2-lymphokine activated killer (LAK) cells in the treatment of primary malignant brain tumors in neuro-oncology. In: Paoletti P et al (eds) Neuro-Oncology. Kluwer Academic Publishers: Developments in Oncology Vol 66, 1991 pp 225-227
80 Papanastassiou V, Pizer BL, Moseley R et al: Target therapy for CNS tumors with monoclonal antibodies. In: Paoletti P et al (eds) Neuro-Oncology. Kluwer Academic Publishers: Developments in Oncology Vol 66, 1991 pp 161-166
81 Kalofonos HP, Pawlikowa TR, Hemingway A et al: Antibody guided diagnosis and therapy of brain glioma using radiolabeled monoclonal antibodies against epidermal growth factor receptor and placental alkaline phosphatase. J Nucl Med 1989 (30):1636-1645
82 Stenning SP, Freedman LS and Bleehen NM: An overview of published results for randomized studies of nitrosoureas in primary high grade malignant glioma. Br J Cancer 1987 (56):89-90
83 Walker M, Alexander E Jr, Hunt W et al: Evaluation of BCNU and/or radiotherapy in the treatment of anaplastic gliomas. A cooperative clinical trial. J Neurosurg 1978 (49): 333-343
84 Afra D, Kocsis B, Dobay J and Eckhardt S: Combined radiotherapy and chemotherapy with dibromodulcitol and CCNU in postoperative treatment of malignant gliomas. J Neurosurg 1983 (59):106-110
85 Scandinavian Glioblastoma Study Group: Combined modality treatment of operated astrocytomas grade 3 and 4. Cancer 1985 (56):41-47
86 Garret MJ, Hughes HJ and Freedman LS: A comparison of radiotherapy alone with radiotherapy and CCNU in cerebral glioma. Clin Oncol 1978 (4):71-79
87 Mahaley MS Jr, Whaley RA, Krigman MR et al: Randomized phase III trial of single versus multiple chemotherapeutic treatment following surgery and during radiotherapy for patients with anaplastic gliomas. Surg Neurol 1987 (27):430-432
88 Eyre HJ, Qualiana JM, Eltringham JR et al: Randomized comparisons of radiation and CCNU versus radiotherapy, CCNU plus procarbazine for treatment of malignant gliomas following surgery. A Southwest Oncology Group report. J Neuro Oncol 1983 (1):171-177
89 Krauseneck P, Messer D, Kleihves P et al: German-Austrian malignant glioma study. Abstracts UICC (Hamburg 1990) p 807
90 Sposto R, Ertel IJ, Jenkin RDT et al: The effectiveness of chemotherapy for treatment of

high grade astrocytoma in children: Results of a randomized trial. J Neuro Oncol 1989 (7):165-177
91 Shapiro WR: Reevaluating the efficacy of intra-arterial BCNU. J Neurosurg 1987 (66):313-315
92 Green SB, Byar DP, Walker MD et al: Comparisons of carmustine, procarbazine and high dose methylprednisolone as additions to surgery and radiotherapy for the treatment of malignant glioma. Cancer Treat Rep 1983 (67):121-132
93 Paoletti P, Butti G and Spanu G: Surgery of cerebral gliomas: State of the art. In: Paoletti P et al (eds) Neuro-Oncology. Kluwer Academic Publishers: Developments in Oncology Vol 66 1991 pp 129-136
94 Di Chiro G: Brain imaging of glucose utilization in cerebral tumours. In: Sokoloff . (ed) Brain Imaging and Brain Function. Raven Press, New York 1985 pp 185-197
95 Chamberlain MC, Murovic J and Levin VA: Absence of contrast enhancement of CT brain scans of patients with supratentorial malignant gliomas. Neurology 1988 (38):1371-1373
96 Tyler JL, Diksic M, Villemure JG et al: Metabolic and hemodynamic evaluation of glioma using positon emission tomography. J Nucl Med 1987 (28):1123-1133
97 Craincross JG and Laperriere NJ: Low-grade glioma. To treat or not to treat. Arch Neurol 1989 (46):1238-1239
98 Soffietti R, Chio A, Giordana MT et al: Prognostic factors in well-differentiated cerebral astrocytomas in the adult. Neurosurgery 1989 (24):686-692
99 Fazekas JT: Treatment of grade I and II brain astrocytomas: the role of radiotherapy. Int J Radiat Oncol Biol Phys 1977 (2):661-666
100 Sheline GE: The role of radiation therapy in the treatment of low-grade gliomas. 35th Annual Congress of Neurological Surgeons. Honolulu, Hawaii, October 1985
101 North CA, North RB, Epstein JA et al: Low-grade cerebral astrocytomas. Survival and quality of life after radiation therapy. Cancer 1990 (66):6-14
102 Ostertag CB: Stereotactic interstitial radiotherapy in the treatment of gliomas. In: Karim ABMF and Laws ER Jr (eds) Glioma: Principles and Practice in Neuro-Oncology. Springer Verlag, Heidelberg 1990
103 Bloom HJG: Management of some intracranial tumours in children and adults. In: Recent Advances in Clinical Oncology. AR Liss Inc, New York 1978 pp 55-84
104 Hildebrand J, Brihaye J, Wagenknecht L et al: Combination chemotherapy with CCNU, vincristine and methotrexate in primary and metastatic brain tumors. Eur J Cancer 1975 (11):585-587
105 Wilkinson IMS, Anderson JR and Holmes AE: Oligodendroglioma: an analysis of 42 cases. J Neurol Neurosurg Psych 1987 (50):304-312
106 Bullard DE, Rawlings CE III, Philips B et al: Oligodendroglioma: an analysis of the value of radiation therapy. Cancer 1987 (60):2179-2188
107 Healy EA, Barnes PD, Kupsky WJ et al: The prognostic significance of post-operative residual tumour in ependymoma. Neurosurgery 1991 (28):666-672
108 Ludwig CL, Smith MT, Bodfrey AD and Armbustmacher VW: A clinicopathological study of 323 patients with oligodendrogliomas. Ann Neurol 1986 19:15-21
109 Bloom HJG and Walsh L: Tumours of the central nervous sytem. In: Bloom HJG et al (eds) Cancer in Children. Clinical Management. Springer-Verlag, Berlin 1975 pp 55-84
110 Cairncross JG and MacDonald DR: Successful chemotherapy for recurrent malignant oligodendroglioma. Ann Neurol 1988 (23):360-364
111 Lyons MK and Kelly PJ: Posterior fossa ependymomas: report of 30 cases and review of the literature. Neurosurgery 1991 (28):659-665
112 Bertolone SJ, Baum ES, Krivit W and Hammond GD: A phase II study of cisplatin therapy in childhood brain tumours. J Neuro Oncol 1989 (7):5-11
113 Sexauer CL, Khan A, Burger PC et al: Cisplatin in recurrent pediatric brain tumours. A POG phase II study. Cancer 1985 (56):1497-1501
114 Khan AB, D'Souza BJ, Wharam MD et al: Cisplatin therapy in recurrent childhood brain tumours. Cancer Treat Rep 1982 (66):2013-2020
115 Tomita T, McLone DG: Medulloblastoma in childhood: results of radical resection and low-dose neuraxis radiation therapy. J Neurosurg 1986 (64):238-42
116 Evans AE, Jenkin RDT, Sposto R et al: Results of a prospective randomized trial of radiation therapy with and without CCNU, vincristine and prednisone. J Neurosurg 1990 (72):572-582
117 Tait DM, Thornton-Jones H, Bloom HJG et al: Adjuvant chemotherapy for medulloblastoma: The first multi-centre control trial of the International Society of Paediatric Oncology (SIOP I). Eur J Cancer 1990 (26):464-469
118 Zucker JM, Mosseri V, Guarnieri S et al: Medulloblastome de l'enfant. L'expérience de l'Institut Curie. Réunion Int Soc Française de Neurologie, June 1991 p 24
119 Walker RW: Medulloblastoma. The Children's Cancer Study Group (CCSG) experience. Réunion Int Soc Française de Neurologie, June 1991 p 25
120 Neidhardt MK (on behalf of the Medulloblastoma Study Committee of the Society of Pediatric Oncology-GPO): Therapeutic approach to medulloblastoma and results: The West German treatment study (interim results). Presented at the 13th International Congress of Chemotherapy, Vienna 1983 (208):29-33
121 Krischer JP, Abdelsalam HR, Kun L et al: Nitrogen mustard, vincristine, procarbazine, and prednisone as adjuvant chemotherapy in the treatment of medulloblastoma. J Neurosurg 1991 (74):905-909
122 Packer RJ, Siegel KR, Sutton LN et al: Efficacy of adjuvant chemotherapy for patients with poor-risk medulloblastoma: a preliminary report. Ann Neurol 1988 (24):503-508
123 McIntosh S, Chen M, Sartain PA et al: Adjuvant chemotherapy for medulloblastoma. Cancer 1985 (56):1316-1319
124 Walker RW, Alleen JC: Cisplatin in the treatment of recurrent childhood primary brain tumours. J Clin Oncol 1988 (6):62-66

125 Chamberlain MC, Prados MD, Silver P and Levin VA: A phase II trial of oral melphalan in recurrent primary brain tumours. Am J Clin Oncol 1988 (11):52-54
126 Allen JC, Helson L: High-dose cyclophosphamide chemotherapy for recurrent CNS tumours in children. J Neurosurg 1981 (55):749-756
127 Duffner PK, Cohen ME: Recent developments in pediatric neuro-oncology. Cancer 1986 (58):561-568
128 Crafts DC, Levin VA, Edwards MS et al: Chemotherapy of recurrent medulloblastomas with combined procarbazine, CCNU and vincristine. J Neurosurg 1978 (49):589-592
129 Lefkowitz IB, Packer RJ, Siegel KR et al Results of treatment of children with recurrent medulloblastoma. Primitive neuroectodermol tumours with lomustine, cisplatin, and vincristine. Cancer 1990 (65):412-417
130 Pendergrass TW, Milstein JM, Geyer RJ et al: Eight drugs in one day chemotherapy for brain tumours: Experience in 107 children and rationale for preradiation chemotherapy. J Clin Oncol 1987 (5):1221-1231
131 Mealey J Jr, Hall PV: Medulloblastoma in children. Survival and treatment. J Neurosurg 1977 (46):56-64
132 Raimondi AJ, Tomita T: Medulloblastoma in childhood. Comparative results of partial and total resection. Childs Brain 1979 (5):310-328
133 Hirsch JF, Renier D, Czernichow P et al: Medulloblastoma in childhood. Survival and functional results. Acta Neurochir 1979 (48):1-15
134 Packer RJ, Sposto R, Atkins TE et al: Quality of life in children with primitive neuroectodermal tumours (medulloblastoma) of the posterior fossa. Pediat. Neurosci 1987 (13):169-175
135 Hochberg FH and Miller C: Primary central nervous system lymphoma. J Neurosurg 1988 (68):835-853
136 De Angelis LM: Primary central nervous system lymphoma. Rev Neurol 1992 (in press)
137 Hochberg FH, Loeffler JS and Prados M The therapy of primary brain lymphoma. J Neuro Oncol 1991 (10):191-201
138 Masson C, Decroix JP, Masson M and Cambier J: Lymphome cérébral primitif. Evolution des données du scanner X sous traitement corticoid. Rev Neurol (Paris) 1985 (141):248-250
139 Henry JM, Heffner RR, Dillard SH et al: Primary malignant lymphomas of the central nervous system. Cancer 1974 (34):1293-1302
140 Bogdhan U, Bogdhan S, Mertens HG et al: Primary non-Hodgkin's lymphomas of the CNS. Acta Neurol Scand 1986 (73):602-614
141 Spaun E, Midholm S, Pedersen NT and Ringsted J: Primary lymphoma of the central nervous system. Surg Neurol 1985 (24):646-650
142 Mendenhall NP, Thar TL, Agee OF et al: Primary lymphoma of the central nervous system. Computerized tomography scan characteristics and treatment results for 12 cases. Cancer 1983 (52):1993-2000
143 Littman P and Wang CC: Reticulum cell sarcoma of the brain. Cancer 1975 (35):1412-1420
144 Kawakami Y, Tabuchi K, Ohnisi T et al: Primary central nervous system lymphoma. J Neurosurg 1985 (62):522-527
145 Letendre L, Banks PM, Reese DR et al: Primary lymphoma of the central nervous system. Cancer 1982 (49):939-943
146 Murray K, Kun L and Cox J: Primary malignant lymphoma of the central nervous system. J Neurosurg 1986 (65):600-607
147 Michalski JM, Garcia DM, Kase E et al: Primary central nervous lymphoma: Analysis of prognostic variables and patterns of treatment failures. Radiology 1990 (176):855-860
148 Allen C, Helson L and Jereb B: Preradiation chemotherapy for newly diagnosed childhood brain tumors. Cancer 1983 (53):2001-2006
149 Horowitz ME, Kun LE, Mulher N et al: Pre-irradiation chemotherapy for brain tumours in children. Neurosurgery 1988 (22):687-690
150 Skarin AT, Zuckerman KS, Pitman SW et al: High dose methotrexate with folinic acid in the treatment of advanced non-Hodgkin's lymphoma including CNS involvement. Blood 1977 (50):1039-1047
151 Griffin J, Thompson RW, Mitchinson MJ et al: Lymphomatous leptomeningitis. Am J Med 1971 (51):200-208
152 Bleyer WA and Griffin TW: White matter necrosis mineralizing microangiopathy, and intellectual abilities in survivors with central nervous system irradiation and methotrexate therapy. In Gilbert HA, Kagan AR (eds) Radiation Damage to the Nervous System. Raven Press, New York 1980 pp 155-174
153 De Angelis LM, Yahalom J, Heinemann MH et al: Primary CNS lymphoma: Combined treatment with chemotherapy and radiotherapy. Neurology 1990 (40):80-86
154 Gabbai AA, Hochberg FH, Linggood R et al: High dose methotrexate therapy of primary brain lymphoma. J Neurosurg 1989 (70):190-194
155 Herbst KD, Corder MP and Justice GR: Successful therapy with methotrexate of a multicentric mixed lymphoma of the central nervous system. Cancer 1976 (38):1476-1478
156 Ervin T and Canellos GP: Successful treatment of recurrent primary central nervous system lymphoma with high dose methotrexate. Cancer 1980 (45):1556-1557
157 Abelson HT, Kufe DW, Skarin AT et al: Treatment of central nervous system tumors with methotrexate. Cancer Treat. Reports 1981 (65):137-140
158 Stewart DJ, Russel N, Dennery M et al: Cyclophosphamide, adriamycin, vincristine and dexamethasone in the treatment of bulky central nervous system lymphomas. J Neuro Oncol 1984 (2):289
159 Shibamoto Y, Tsutsui K, Dodo Y et al: Improved survival rate in primary intracranial lymphoma treated by high-dose radiation and systemic vincristine - doxorubicin - cyclophosphamide - prednisolone chemotherapy. Cancer 1990 (65):1907-1912
160 Cohen IJ, Vogel R, Matz S et al: Successful non-neurotoxic therapy (without radiation) of a multifocal primary brain lymphoma with

methotrexate, vincristine, and BCNU. Protocol (DEMOB) Cancer 1986 (57):6-11
161 McLaughlin P, Velasques WS, Redman JR et al: Chemotherapy with dexamethasone, high-dose cytarabine, and cisplatin for parenchymal brain lymphoma. JNCI 1988 (80):1408-1412
162 Remick SC, Diamond C, Migliozzi JA et al: Primary central nervous system lymphoma in patients with and without the acquired immune deficiency syndrome. Medicine 1990 (69):345-360

Treatment of Brain Metastases

Khê Hoang-Xuân and Jean-Yves Delattre

Service de Neurologie, Hôpital de la Salpêtrière, Boulevard de l'Hôpital 47, 75013 Paris, France

Intracranial metastasis is a common complication of systemic cancer occuring in 25% of patients; two-thirds of these lesions are parenchymal cerebral metastases. Lung and breast represent approximately 50% of primary tumours. Melanoma, cancer of the kidney and digestive tract are the next common causes of brain metastasis. In 20% of cases the primary tumour remains unknown. In most series about 30% of patients have single and 70% multiple brain metastases. Brain metastases of malignant melanoma and lung cancer are usually multiple. Except for brain metastases from primary lung tumours, cerebral metastases are late events in the course of a cancer; two-thirds of patients have extracranial metastasis at time of diagnosis, mainly lung metastasis. Brain metastases are rarely the first manifestation of cancer. The clinical presentation of brain metastasis includes an acute onset (50%) with seizures and pseudovascular deficits. This last mode of onset may reflect bleeding in the metastatic lesion, tumour embolism, cystic transformation or tumoural necrosis. The clinical presentation can also be progressive (50%) with symptoms of intracranial hypertension, neurological deficits and disturbance of consciousness. The symptoms are due to the tumour itself and to the vasogenic peritumoural oedema. CT and MRI of the head with contrast are highly sensitive methods to detect brain metastasis in cancer patients. However, the radiologic appearence of the lesions is not specific. In a recent study, 10% of suspected brain metastases on the basis of scans were not confirmed at cerebral biopsy. Therefore, a pathologic diagnosis is indicated if the primary tumour is unknown and sometimes also if the primary tumour is known but the nature of the intracranial lesion is dubious (long delay between diagnosis of the cancer and first symptoms of brain metastasis, infectious context).

If not treated, patients suffering from brain metastases have a median survival of about 1 month [1]. The treatment of brain metastases is still essentially palliative. Its aim is to increase the patient's survival if possible but above all to preserve the quality of the remaining life by limiting or improving the neurological symptoms which might impair it.

The data given in articles on the treatment of brain metastases are difficult to interpret for several reasons:

1) Almost all reported studies are retrospective and their results are therefore subject to many kinds of bias.

2) Primary cancers are almost always grouped together, although the sensitivity of brain metastases to different forms of treatment varies with the nature of the primary cancer. Moreover, patients received several forms of treatment which makes it very difficult to know which of them was effective.

3) The cause of death (neurological or systemic) is often unknown, although this datum is essential for judging the effectiveness of treatment of the brain metastases.

The various criteria for evaluating the effectiveness of treatment are difficult to interpret because they are not specific enough.

1) Median survival, the traditional index used in the studies, is much more an indication of the spread of the primary cancer. Indeed, most studies agree that more patients die from systemic complications than as a direct result of their brain metastases [2]. Moreover, median survival takes no account of the qual-

ity of survival which is still the main aim of the treatment.
2) The development of neurological symptoms can be deceptive. Apart from their subjective nature, they are extremely sensitive to corticoids which makes it difficult to evaluate associated treatments. On the other hand, the worsening or reappearance of neurological symptoms does not always mean that the tumour has progressed or recurred. The symptoms may result from a metabolic encephalopathy frequent in advanced cancer cases, or from a vascular complication (nonbacterial thrombotic endocarditis, DIC) or a brain infection taking advantage of immunosuppression (meningitis, cerebral abscess, fungal infection or any other opportunistic infection). Finally, delayed complications from radiotherapy or chemotherapy may simulate a recurrent tumour.
3) CT scan and MRI of the brain are the most objective criteria for evaluation. However, they also cause problems of interpretation (it is not always easy to distinguish between radionecrosis and recurrence of the tumour; between a response to a specific treatment and reduced contrast merely resulting from corticotherapy). In the case of surgical resection, the first post-operative CT-scan should be carried out between 48 and 72 hours after the operation to avoid secondary contrast enhancement related to surgical manipulation.
4) Lastly, the duration of response to treatment can be assessed only in patients whose neurological lesions develop more quickly than the systemic cancer.
Corticotherapy, antiepileptics, surgery, radiotherapy and chemotherapy are used.

Glucocortocoids

Dexamethasone and methylprednisolone are the most commonly used, the latter producing less muscular toxicity. They often have a spectacular, rapid effect (within hours or, more often, days). The usual dosage is 16 mg of dexamethasone per day and 80 mg of methylprednisolone per day. If necessary, doses of dexamethasone may be increased to 100 mg and doses of methylprednisolone to 500 mg. Over 70% of patients improve clinically [3] and the scanner shows reduction of contrast enhancement and brain oedema. However, glucocorticoids have only a transitory effect and there is little change in median survival when corticotherapy is used alone (2 months). Glucocorticoids reduce the vasogenic brain oedema (by reducing capillary permeability in the blood-tumour barrier and probably by speeding up reabsorption of the oedema already formed); they do not have an oncolytic effect on carcinomas [4]. They are usually given in conjunction with radiotherapy as they improve the patient's tolerance of the therapy. Because of their long-term side effects (myopathy, diabetes, hypercatabolism), they must be gradually tapered as the patient's clinical condition improves after radiotherapy and surgery.

Antiepileptics

In 6-29% of cases, an epileptic seizure is the first symptom of brain metastases. About 10% more patients have epileptic seizures in the course of the disease [5]. Antiepileptic treament must be prescribed systematically for these patients. The treatment is also recommended just after surgical resection of the tumour but it should probably not be prolonged if the patient has never had a seizure. Antiepileptics can have many side effects. Thus, administering diphenylhydantoin or carbamazepine in conjunction with brain radiation therapy seems to increase the risk of a skin reaction in the irradiated area, which can develop into a sometimes fatal Stevens-Johnson syndrome [6,7]. Phenobarbital is responsible for a shoulder-hand syndrome (algodystrophy) in over 10% of patients suffering from a brain tumour. In addition, antiepileptics reduce the bioavailability of corticoids and their enzyme-inductive effect may affect the metabolism of chemotherapeutic drugs. Among patients who had not previously had an epileptic seizure, it has not been shown that untreated patients later had more seizures than those who had been given preventive treatment [5]. Therefore, it is generally not advised to prescribe prophylactic antiepileptics systematically for patients suffering from brain metastases who have never had an epileptic seizure. The sole exception is in the case of brain metastases from melanomas which cause twice as many seizures as other brain metastases. In a study on brain metastases from melanomas, Hagen [8] showed that systematically prescribing antiepileptics reduced the risk of later seizures by a factor of 2. The highly epileptogenic nature of these brain metastases is related to the fact that they are usually located in the grey matter.

Surgery

Surgical excision has several advantages [9]:
a) it enables a histological diagnosis to be made;
b) it produces an immediate decompressive effect by reducing the size of the tumour and its accompanying brain oedema;
c) it thus facilitates the action of radiotherapy;
d) it can induce long periods of remission or even cure the disease [10].
Generally, surgery is suggested for only a limited number patients who fulfil the following conditions:
a) the tumour must be located at a single, accessible site in the brain;
b) the primary tumour must be in remission or under control;
c) there must not be any other metastatic sites;
d) the patient must be in good general condition.
However, surgery is sometimes envisaged under special circumstances:
a) When the primary cancer is developing, if there is a chance that it can be controlled while the brain metastasis is being treated. Epidermoid carcinomas and pulmonary adenocarcinomas in advanced stages which exhibit a single brain metastasis with no other metastatic sites respond well to a craniotomy followed by brain radiotherapy in conjunction with thoracic radiotherapy and polychemotherapy. Long-term survival is obtained in one-third of such cases with a median survival of 12 to 26 months [11]. Choriocarcinomas, even when there are other metastatic sites, respond very well to effective chemotherapy [12]; however, excision of a brain metastasis which, by bleeding, may have had an adverse effect on the vital prognosis, is sometimes useful [12].
b) Excision of multiple brain metastases can sometimes be carried out simultaneously or successively at 2 or 3 sites, provided they are all accessible.
c) When there is systemic spread of the primary tumour, surgical removal of a brain metastasis, while not curative, can sometimes improve the quality of life and give medical treatment (especially chemotherapy) time to act on the systemic sites.
In practice, if surgery is possible it is often chosen when extracranial metastatic sites are not immediately threatening, allowing the patient to hope for more than 3 to 4 months of good-quality survival, which is the average neurological remission after radiotherapy alone.
Surgical mortality has improved markedly in recent years and is currently about 5% [13]. A similar mortality is observed in the first month following RT [13]. Median survival ranges from 6 to 10 months after the operation and 25% to 43% of patients observed in the main studies (Table 1) are still alive a year later.

Table 1. Surgery for single brain metastases

Series	Year	No.pts.	Postop. mortality	Median survival (months)	1-year survival	Long-term survival
Raskin [72]	1971	51	12%	6	30%	10% (3y)
Haar [73]	1972	167	11%	6	22%	5% (5y)
Ransohoff [74]	1975	100	10%	6	38%	13% (2y)
Galicich [15]	1980	78	4,8,32%*	6	29%	-
Winston [75]	1980	79	10%	5	22%	10% (2y)
White [14]	1981	122	6%	7	30%	15% (2y)
Patchell [16]	1990	25	4%	10	42%	0%

* Neurological grades I, II and III, respectively

Several prognostic factors can influence survival:
a) the histological nature of the primary tumour [14];
b) the patient's neurological condition at the time of surgery. In the series of Galicich et al. [15], 1-year survival was 44% among patients with no major motor deficiency whereas it was only 11% among deficient patients;
c) when the interval between the diagnosis of the primary cancer and the appearance of brain metastases is greater than 1 year, it seems to correlate with a better prognosis [15]. Median survival rises from 4 to 7 months and 1-year survival from 19% to 36% if the brain metastases are discovered more than a year after the primary cancer. This correlation could indicate the tumour's rate of development and the host's defensive reactions to it;
d) localisation within the brain. The prognosis for infratentorial metastases is not as good. In the series of White et al. [14], two-thirds of the patients who died within 2 months after the operation had a subtentorial tumour;
e) age;
f) the extent of surgery (complete versus partial removal);
g) systemic extension at the time of the craniotomy is a factor of poor prognosis in several studies [16,17].

Radiotherapy

Methods

Conventional radiotherapy

The usual sources of radiation are telecobalt and linear accelerators. The irradiation field generally includes the whole brain because multiple brain metastases are frequent. Even in the case of a single metastasis, most authors recommend whole-brain irradiation in the hope that it will destroy microscopic foci of metastases that are not seen on CT or MRI. Doses usually vary between 30 and 40 Gy, in fractions of 2 or 3 Gy a day. Randomised studies comparing various protocols ranging from 20 Gy delivered in 1 week (5 fractions) to 40 Gy in 4 weeks (20 fractions) did not show a greater palliative effect for any treatment schedule in particular, even on a subgroup of patients with a more favourable prognosis [18-20]. Some authors have advised concentrating the treatment to make it shorter (10 Gy in 1 fraction or 15 Gy in 2 fractions over 3 days), thus making the treatment less restrictive for the patients. However, these protocols are no longer recommended because they are associated with a higher early death rate and side effects (signs of increased intracranial hypertension due to oedema) [21]. When predicted survival exceeds 1 year, particularly after surgery, we use a dose of 45 Gy delivered in fractions of 1.8 Gy, in order to reduce the risk of delayed radiation-induced dementia which can be observed in 10% to 20% of long-term survivors [22]. If the systemic or local extension of the cancer makes death within 6 months likely, we irradiate the whole brain with a dose of 30 Gy in 10 fractions over 15 days. Parenteral corticotherapy is systematically prescribed during irradiation. Prophylactic brain radiotherapy, used mainly for small cell lung cancers, is discussed below.

Stereotactic radiotherapy

Brain radiotherapy has benefitted in recent years from remarkable progress made in medical imaging (scanner, MRI) which can now provide a 3-dimensional reconstruction of the tumour. Interstitial radiotherapy and external stereotactic radiotherapy now enable irradiation to be very precisely targeted.

Interstitial radiotherapy (brachytherapy)

Interstitial radiotherapy is a stereotactic technique using catheters to implant one or several radioactive sources in the tumour. They are inserted externally under anaesthetic and scanner control. Iodine 125 is most commonly used because its low energy emission in the form of gamma and X-rays enables healthy tissue next to the tumour to be preserved. The dose delivered to the tumour is about 0.5 Gy an hour. The radioactive source can be removed once the desired dose has been delivered (usually 4 to 6 days later). The usual doses range from 30 to 120 Gy [23]. Interstitial radiotherapy has several advantages over conventional radiotherapy. It enables high doses of irradiation to be delivered electively to the site of the tumour while sparing the rest of the brain. It can also be used with conventional radiotherapy to give a local boost. Interstitial radiotherapy can also be used in conjunction with interstitial hyperthermia which has an oncolytic effect (radiothermy) [24,25]. The main side effect is the high incidence of focal radionecrosis, causing brain oedema, which requires surgical resection of the necrotic focus 6 to 8 months following implant in about half of the cases. Radionecrosis may cause diagnostic difficulties because both under clinical examination and on the scanner it may resemble a recurrent tumour.

External stereotactic radiotherapy (ESR)

External stereotactic radiotherapy differs from interstitial radiotherapy in several ways [26]:
A radioactive source is not implanted in the parenchyma of the brain. Irradiation is usually delivered by a modified linear accelerator, but other sources of radiation have been used (helium, protons, gamma unit) [27]. The dose is delivered to the target by intersection of the beams in its centre; the beams enter through a large number of points spread over the surface of the scalp. Thus, external stereotactic radiotherapy concentrates irradiation mainly in the tumour while sparing the contiguous tissues.
It can be used for very small lesions (1 cm^3) and for sites in which it is difficult to implant iodine 125, even with stereotaxy.
Treatment is given in a single 10-30 Gy fraction. Patients therefore find it less restricting. Symptomatic radionecrosis seems less frequent.

Indications

Indications are currently limited to clearly definable single tumours, with a diameter of less than 6 cm for interstitial radiotherapy and less than 3 cm for external stereotactic radiotherapy (23,24,26,28). Tumours must also be supratentorial for interstitial radiotherapy but there are exceptions to this rule. Interstitial radiotherapy and external stereotactic radiotherapy are currently used to treat recurrent brain metastases after conventional radiotherapy has failed, but their indication may be extended to include treatment of brain metastases by first intention in conjunction with whole brain radiotherapy [28].

Results

Conventional Radiotherapy

Radiotherapy is still the preferred treatment for brain metastases. Its role is essentially palliative, however, on very rare occasions can it be curative. After studying post-mortem neuropathological examinations performed on a series of 187 patients treated with radiotherapy for brain metastases, Cairncross found complete sterilisation had occurred in 3% of the cases [29]. In most studies, between 2/3 and 3/4 of the patients respond well to radiotherapy [2] (Table 2). In some studies treatment responses vary, depending on the histological nature of the tumours and on whether or not the studies included patients who died in the course of treatment. Improvements generally last an average of only 3 months and the median survival is between 3 and 6 months [2]. Only 10-20% of patients are still alive a year later (Table 2). As already remarked, median survival is not a good indication of the value of the treatment because the cause of death is frequently systemic. Nearly 60% of the patients who are alive 6 months after radiotherapy still show neurological improvement [2,30]. The best criteria for evaluating patient response to radiotherapy are CT-scan of the brain and whether or not corticotherapy needs to be maintained. Cairncross and Posner [2] evaluated their patients' response to radiotherapy by using the CT scanner. Although the median survival of about 3 months was similar to previous studies, they observed that the brain metastases had become much smaller or had disappeared in 60% of cases. The neurological improvement observed at the same time continued until the patient's death, caused by extracranial metastatic sites in two-thirds of the cases. In only one-third of cases was death directly attributable to brain metastases or due to both neurological and systemic causes.

Table 2. Radiotherapy for brain metastases

Series	Year	No.pts.	RT / protocol	Response	Median survival (months)	1-year survival
Young [21]	1974	83*	15 Gy / 2 fr / 3 days	57%	2	-
		79	30 Gy / 3 weeks	62%	4	-
Berry [76]	1974	124*	variable	63%	4	10%
Hendrickson [19]	1977	1001	10 Gy / 1 fr to 40 Gy / 3 weeks	52%	4	15%
Markesbery [77]	1978	129	30 Gy / 3 weeks	-	4	12%
Cairncross [2]	1980	183	39 Gy / 17 days	78%	3	8%
Zimm [17]	1981	156	variable	-	3	12%
Patchell [16]	1990	23	36 Gy / 12 fr / 2 weeks	-	4	10%

* including operated patients

Stereotactic radiotherapy

The use of interstitial radiotherapy and external stereotactic radiotherapy in the treatment of brain metastases is still in the experimental phase. Because only a limited number of selected patients are treated, it is difficult to compare the results obtained with results produced by other forms of treatment. Early reports are nonetheless encouraging, both for initial treatment of brain metastasis and for recurrent cases (see "Treatment of Recurrent Brain Metastases").

As a treatment primarily aimed at brain metastases, Sturm [31] used external stereotactic radiotherapy from the outset on 12 patients exhibiting radioresistant, inoperable brain metastases. With the exception of 1 patient who died less than 24 hours after being given external stereotactic radiotherapy, all patients improved clinically and radiologically with remissions ranging from 3 to 9 months at the end of the study. Prados [28] treated 4 patients with conventional radiotherapy followed 2 weeks later by an interstitial radiotherapeutic boost. One of the patients died a month later from extracranial metastatic complications of the cancer, although he was in good neurological condition. The 3 others were still alive at the end of the study with 13 months' survival for 2 patients and 21 months' survival for the third. Marin-Grez [32] used the same protocol and obtained a complete or partial response in 11 out of 26 patients and stabilisation in 13 patients.

Further studies should give a better indication of the optimal dose to be delivered, the quality of long-term survival, the frequency of symptomatic radionecrosis and the subgroups of brain metastases most likely to benefit from the treatment. Such studies should also compare the effectiveness of stereotactic radiotherapy with the effectiveness of surgery both in the initial treatment and in treatment of recurrent, operable brain metastases. Technical improvements now enable external stereotactic radiotherapy to be administered in several fractions [33].

Prophylactic Brain Radiotherapy

This technique is used for lung cancers, mainly small cell lung cancers. The usual dose is 30 Gy in fractions of 3 Gy over 2 weeks and should be administered as soon as possible after chemotherapy has finished [34]. Some authors have suggested increasing the dosage because they believe that the recurrence of brain tumours after preventive brain radiotherapy is due to insufficient initial sterilisation rather than a new spreading process [35]. Several randomised prospective studies on small cell lung cancer have shown that prophylactic brain radiotherapy reduces the frequency of brain metastases from 23% to 5% [36]. However, prophylactic brain radiotherapy does not alter the median survival because patients frequently die from systemic extension of the primary tumour. Opinions differ on the systematic use of prophylactic brain radiotherapy. Some authors found that most neurological symptoms regressed when radiotherapy was administered at the time the brain metastases appeared [37]. In addition, they believed that preventive brain radiotherapy did not prevent the formation of new sites within the brain [36]; lastly, prophylactic brain radiotherapy exposed patients to a substantial risk of cerebral toxicity. It is estimated that 10-60% of the patients who survive for a year or more after prophylactic brain radiotherapy develop cognitive disorders. For that reason, some authors suggest to reduce the dose and not to administer brain radiotherapy during chemotherapy, in an effort to reduce combined toxic effects [38,39]. Most authors recommend prophylactic RT only when there is complete remission of the lung cancer. In addition, it was recently suggested to use a lower dose (25 Gy in 10 fractions of 2.5 Gy) and to administer RT only after completion of chemotherapy [38].

Prophylactic brain radiotherapy apparently also reduces the incidence of brain metastases from other lung cancers [40], particularly adenocarcinomas [41]. Indications are limited to lung cancers in remission and those with local involvement of the lymph nodes N1-N2, which increase the risk of brain metastases by a factor of 4 or 5 [41]. The dosage and radiotherapeutic methods used are the same as for small cell lung cancer.

Chemotherapy

Chemotherapy has long taken a second place in the treatment of brain metastases. It does, however, have the advantage of being able to act simultaneously on brain metastases and on the other systemic sites. Chemotherapy has mostly been used as an adjuvant to radiotherapy and its effectiveness is therefore difficult to assess. Moreover, the protocols used varied from one study to another and sometimes within the same study. The main theoretical difficulty of chemotherapy is the crossing of the blood-brain barrier which lets through only small molecules or liposoluble products. The blood-brain barrier is a real obstacle for small brain metastases which have not yet induced abundant neovascularisation. This fact is well illustrated in experiments by Ushio [42], who showed that injecting cells of the Walker 256 carcinoma into the common carotid artery of rats led to the development of metastases in the area of the external (maxillary) and the internal (cerebral) carotid arteries. Shortly after the malignant cells had been injected, chemotherapy was administered using cyclophosphamide (very little of which passes through the normal blood-brain barrier): the development of the maxillary metastases was inhibited while the brain metastases continued to grow. These results showed that an insufficient amount of the drug had reached the micrometastases in the brain because of the blood-brain barrier. The problem is more complicated when the brain metastases cause neovascularisation composed of fenestrated capillaries with little or no barrier properties, as illustrated by the contrast enhancement in the tumour on the CT scanner. Pharmacokinetic studies have shown that molecules such as methotrexate, 5-FU, bleomycin and cyclophosphamide, in spite of being water-soluble, can reach the tumour site in sufficient amounts to produce a cytotoxic effect [43]. However, it has not been established whether or not a sufficient concentration of water-soluble cytotoxic agents can reach the brain around the tumour, which is partly invaded by tumoural cells but still has most of its barrier properties. Nitrosourea derivatives (BCNU, CCNU, ACNU) have been most often used. They were moderately effective with a response rate of about 20% limited to a few months [44]. Intra-arterial chemotherapy using BCNU or cisplatin has not proved to be better than the intravenous method (response rate of 20-50%, median survival 4 months) [45-47]. Recently, other chemotherapeutic protocols have been used as first-line treatment for brain metastases from lung and breast cancers, with encouraging results [43,48,49] (Table 3). The most important study was carried out by Rosner [43] who treated 100 patients with brain metastases from breast cancer with 4 different chemotherapeutic protocols. He obtained a partial or complete response from half of the patients with a median survival of 5.5 months (Table 3). It is worth noting that 17 out of 19 patients who were given radiotherapy after chemotherapy had failed did not respond, suggesting that the development of resis-

Table 3. Chemotherapy for brain metastases

Series	Year	Cancer	No. pts	Protocol	Response	Median survival (months)	1-year survival
Hildebrand [78]	1975	Breast	11	CCNU, M, V	45%	-	-
Rosner [43]	1986	Breast	100	CFP ± MV MVP CA	50%	5.5	31%
Cocconi [50]	1990	Breast	22	CDDP, VP16	55%	14*	55%
Kleisbauer [62]	1988	SCLC NSCLC	13	VP16	30%	2.5	-
Postmus [49]	1989	SCLC	23	VP16	43%	-	-
Twelves [79]	1990	SCLC	19	C, V, VP16	53%	7*	20%
Lee [55]	1990	SCLC	11	C, A, V, VP16	82%	8**	-
Kleisbauer [80]	1990	SCLC NSCLC	24	CDDP	30%	3.5*	12%
Thomas [53]	1990	SCLC NSCLC	60	VP16 CDDP	30%	3	-
Robinet [52]	1991	SCLC NSCLC	16	CDDP, F	50%	9	30%
Jacquillat [51]	1990	Melanoma	39	Fotemustine	28%	6.5	21%

* including patients treated with radiotherapy while in remission or after failure of therapy
** chemotherapy associated with radiotherapy as primary treatment modality
SCLC = small cell lung cancer; NSCLC = non-small cell lung cancer
M = methotrexate; V = vincristine; C = cyclophosphamide; F = 5-fluorouracil; P = prednisone; A = adriamycin
VP16 = etoposide; CDDP = cisplatin

tance to chemotherapy also induces resistance to brain radiotherapy. Other protocols are currently being assessed, e.g., VP16 and cisplatin for breast and lung cancer and fotemustine for melanomas [50-53]. In rare cases, chemotherapy may "cure" brain metastases. Thus, Rustin [12] treated with chemotherapy 18 patients suffering from brain metastases from choriocarcinoma. The protocol alternated methotrexate-VP16-dactinomycin and cyclophosphamide-vincristine. Thirteen patients (72%) went into full remission with a median follow-up treatment of 33 months. The role of chemotherapy in the treatment of brain metastases therefore deserves to be re-evaluated. There has not yet been a controlled study comparing the effectiveness of radiotherapy in conjunction with chemotherapy with the effectiveness of radiotherapy alone as initial treatment of brain metastases. A retrospective study [54] suggested that the former therapeutic strategy was more effective in terms of survival (8.3 months versus 4.3 months).

Therapeutic Indications

Signs of intracranial hypertension and tentorial herniation require emergency treatment including high doses of corticoids, osmotic agents and even hyperventilation.

Radiotherapy is not recommended on an emergency basis because it may aggravate the brain oedema; it is more appropriate to start RT when the neurological condition of the patient has been improved following 48-72 hours of high-dose corticoids. Emergency surgery is indicated only in the case of intracranial hypertension caused by hydrocephalus to provide ventricular drainage. Apart from this special case, the choice of treatment is governed by 3 parameters (see algorythm):

1) The nature of the primary cancer, which largely influences sensitivity to treatment. Thus, brain metastases from choriocarcinoma can be cured by chemotherapy while a brain metastasis from cancer of the colon or kidney is often resistant to both radiotherapy and chemotherapy.

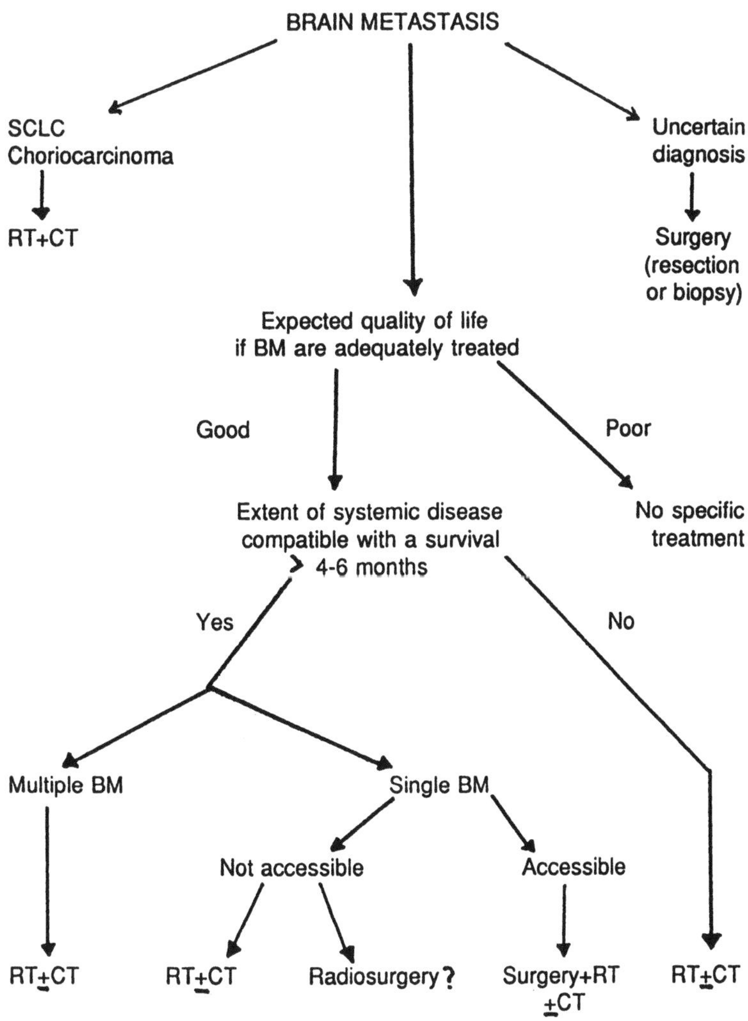

BM: brain metastasis
SCLC: small cell lung cancer
RT: radiotherapy
CT: chemotherapy

2) Neurological examination. The functional condition of the patient at the beginning of the treatment is an important prognostic factor both for the amount and the quality of remaining life. CT-scanning and, more recently, MRI following infusion of gadolinium localises brain metastatic sites and specifies their number. As a general rule, surgery is considered only when there is a single brain metastasis. Whenever possible, a lumbar puncture is made to test for associated carcinomatous meningitis, because the presence of this disease would influence the treatment schedule.

3) Systemic examination takes into account non-specific factors such as age and diathesis as well as specific factors related to the metastatic spread of the cancer. The search for other metastases (pulmonary, hepatic, osseous) should be systematic and is positive in nearly 75% of cases. Analysis of the systemic extension of the cancer enables predictions to be made about the patient's life expectancy and potential quality of life if the brain metastases are properly treated. Thus, although it seldom happens, the clinician may decide not to treat the brain metastases when they occur in a patient suffering severe, persistent pain related to systemic, untreatable extension of the cancer. Under these circumstances, the disturbances of the patient's wakefulness which rapidly result from spon-

Table 4. Surgery + RT vs RT alone for single brain metastasis

Series	Year	Cancer	No. pts. (RT/S + RT)	Median survival RT	Median survival S + RT	1-year survival RT	1-year survival S + RT
Mandell [61]	1986	NSCLC	69 / 35	4	16	30%	66%
Patchell [57]	1986	NSCLC	43 / 43	9	19	37%	65%
Patchell [16]	1990	All types	23 / 25	4	10	10%	42%

RT = radiotherapy; S = surgery

taneous development of brain metastases are not interfered with. In the other cases, the brain metastases should be treated.

When extracranial metastatic spread is developing rapidly, the treatment is simply palliative and surgery is contraindicated. If the cancer is under control and the patient is in good general condition, a more radical, curative treatment may be attempted.

Recent work by Patchell et al. [16] suggests that surgical resection should be proposed to treat a single, surgically accessible brain metastasis, except in the case of primaries which are highly sensitive to radio or chemotherapy (such as small cell lung cancer or choriocarcinoma) (Table 4). Since no prospective randomised study has been conducted it is not clearly established that radiotherapy is necessary after complete excision of a brain metastasis. Nevertheless, two retrospective studies suggest that post-operative radiotherapy delays or lessens the risk of neurological recurrences, although it does not modify median survival [8,56]. Another solution is to begin the treatment with radiotherapy and to reserve resection for patients who do not respond or who relapse. One retrospective study suggests that this strategy is unsatisfactory [57], perhaps because radiotherapy is more effective on small tumours and in particular on residual, post-operative lesions [57].

When surgical excision is inappropriate, i.e., in about 80% of cases, the choice of treatment is relatively simple. In these cases, brain radiotherapy is indicated - perhaps in conjunction with chemotherapy. Brain radiotherapy is used to treat most multiple brain metastases, as well as single, inaccessible brain metastases and single brain metastases associated with an uncontrollable, spreading primary tumour or with other metastatic sites which constitute a short-term threat.

Treatment of Recurrent Metastases

There are several ways to treat a brain metastasis which recurs after surgery. Their indications have not yet been fully defined.

Reoperation

Surgically removed brain metastases recur locally in about one-third of patients; two-thirds of these patients are candidates for reoperation. Reoperating is an effective measure: in over two-thirds of the cases it leads to neurological improvement lasting an average of 6 months. Median survival is 9 months after the second operation [58] and 1 out of 4 patients is still alive a year later. For these selected patients, therefore, the results are comparable to the results of the first operation.

Further Radiation Treatment

Further radiation treatment is indicated in some instances (sometimes in conjunction with chemotherapy) when reoperation is not. The dosage is usually from 20 to 25 Gy in 10 fractions [59] with response rates ranging from 27% to 75%, depending on the study [59,60] and a median survival from 2 to 5 months after the new irradiation. Further irradiation benefits only patients in good general condition who responded well to initial radiotherapy, with an improvement which lasts over 4 months [59].

Stereotactic Radiotherapy

Prados [28] gave stereotactic radiotherapy treatment to 10 patients (in 9 of whom conventional radiotherapy had already failed). Median survival was 20 months; 5 patients died (after an average 5-month survival). Death was attributed to both recurrence of the brain metastases and spread of the cancer in 3 cases; to recurrent brain metastases alone in 1 case (but the patient died more than 2 years after interstitial radiotherapy), and to cancer spread in 1 case. Seven patients were still alive 1 year later. Loeffler [26] used external stereotactic radiotherapy to treat 20 patients who had not responded to conventional radiotherapy or who had subsequently relapsed. In all of them, the brain metastases were stabilised or reduced, with an average remission of 9 months, except for 2 patients who were later successfully treated by surgical excision and interstitial radiotherapy. The treatment was used again on 1 patient who developed a brain metastasis at a distant site. Brain metastases from adenocarcinoma seem to respond much more quickly (less than 6 weeks) than metastases from melanomas or sarcomas which more often stabilise. No case of symptomatic radionecrosis was reported.

Chemotherapy

Former treatment does not seem to affect the response of brain metastases to chemotherapy. In a study by Rosner [43], 3 of the 4 patients in whom radiotherapy had failed responded to chemotherapy. Furthermore, 37% of the patients who relapsed after a first chemotherapeutic protocol responded to a second chemotherapy treatment.

Treatment of Brain Metastases from Lung Cancer

Brain metastases from a primary lung cancer generally have a very poor prognosis. Single, accessible brain metastases (with the exception of small cell cancers) must be operated. Retrospective studies by Mandell et al. [61] and Patchell et al. [57] showed a significantly higher median survival among patients treated by surgery in conjunction with radiotherapy compared with patients treated by radiotherapy alone (Table 4). Survival was thus extended by 10 months (19 versus 9 months).

Brain metastases respond to radiotherapy in about two-thirds of cases but survival remains low and varies between 3 and 6 months in the main studies (Table 4). A study by Carmichael [36] on brain metastases from small cell lung cancer suggests that the duration of response in patients who survive the first 2 months increases with the dose delivered. Thus, the response lasted for 10 months when the dose delivered was higher than 40 Gy while it lasted only 5 months when the dose was between 30 and 40 Gy.

Several chemotherapeutic protocols prescribed as first-line treatment have recently given encouraging results (median survival varying between 3 and 9 months) with good haematologic tolerance (cyclophosphamide-vincristine-adriamycin-VP16; cisplatin-5FU; cisplatin; VP16) (Table 5). A high dose of VP16 (1500 mg/m^2) gives responses in 30% to 40% of the cases but is complicated by bone marrow aplasia (almost always fatal) in half of the cases [49,62,63]. An uncontrolled retrospective study by Takakura [54] suggests that radiotherapy in conjunction with chemotherapy gives longer survival rates than radiotherapy alone (6.7 versus 3.4 months) (Fig. 1).

Treatment of Brain Metastases from Breast Cancer

Brain metastases originating from the breast respond to radiotherapy in 50% to 70% of cases. Median survival varies from 3 to 6 months after irradiation. According to Takakura et al., median survival after surgery alone is 5 months and 12 months when surgical excision is followed by radiotherapy (Table 6). However, the advantage of radiotherapy after surgery has not been clearly

Table 5. Treatment of brain metastases from lung cancer

Series	Year	No. pts.	Treatment	Protocol	Response	Median surv. (months)	1-year survival
Deeley [81]	1968	61	RT	30 Gy / 4 weeks	47%	6	14%
Horton [82]	1971	19	RT	40 Gy / 3-4 weeks	74%	5	-
Montana [83]	1972	47	RT	variable	56%	3.5	10%
Hazra [84]	1972	25	RT	40 Gy / 3 weeks	76%	5	12%
Gilbert [85]	1979	55	RT	13 Gy / 2 days	50%	3-6	-
Nugent [86]	1979	51*	RT	variable	92%	3	-
Cairncross [2]	1980	68	RT	39 Gy / 17 days	80%	3	7%
Takakura [54]	1981	51	RT	variable	-	3-5	8%
Mandell [61]	1986	69	RT	variable	72%	4	18%
Patchell [57]	1986	43	RT	variable	83%	9	37%
Carmichael [36]	1988	59*	RT	30-40 Gy	63%	3-7	37%
Montana [83]	1972	15	S	-	-	6	-
White [14]	1981	38	S	-	-	6	11%
Takakura [54]	1981	64	S	-	-	5	-
Takakura [54]	1981	51	S+RT	-	-	11	-
Mandell [61]	1986	35	S+RT	-	-	16	66%
Patchell [57]	1986	43	S+RT	-	-	19	65%
Twelves [79]	1990	19*	C	**C**, V, VP16	53%	7	20%
Lee [55]	1990	11*	C	**C**, A, V, VP16	82%	8	-
Kleisbauer [80]	1990	24	C	CDDP	30%	3.5	12%
Thomas [53]	1990	60	C	CDDP; VP16	30%	3	-
Robinet [52]	1991	16	C	CDDP, F	50%	9	30%

* SCLC only
RT = radiotherapy; S = surgery; C = chemotherapy; **C** = cyclophosphamide; V = vincristine; A = adriamycin; VP16 = etoposide; CDDP = cisplatin; F = 5-fluorouracil

shown in a prospective randomised study. Chemotherapy has recently been used as first-line treatment in 2 studies, one by Rosner and one by Cocconi [43,50], with a response rate of about 50% and a median survival of 5.5 months and 14 months, respectively (Table 6). In the Rosner series, one-third of the patients who had relapsed responded to

Table 6. Treatment of brain metastases from breast cancer

Series	Year	No. pts.	Treatment	Protocol	Response	Median survival (months)	1-year survival
Gilbert [83]	1979	21	RT	20 Gy / 1 week	50%	3-7	-
Di Stefano [87]	1979	87	RT	variable	-	4	-
Cairncross [2]	1980	37	RT	39 Gy / 17 days	75%	3	22%
Takakura [54]	1981	21	S	-	-	5	23%
Takakura [54]	1981	11	S+RT	-	-	12	
Rosner [43]	1986	100	C	CFP ± MV; MVP; **C**A	50%	5.5	15%
Cocconi [50]	1990	22	C	VP16, CDDP	55%	14	55%
Lange [88]	1990	61	C+RT	Ifos, BCNU 45 Gy / fr 1.5 Gy	65%	8	-

RT = radiotherapy; S = surgery; C = chemotherapy
C = cyclophosphamide; F = 5-fluorouracil; P = prednisone; M = methotrexate; V = vincristine; A = adriamycin; VP16 = etoposide; CDDP = cisplatin; Ifos = ifosfamide

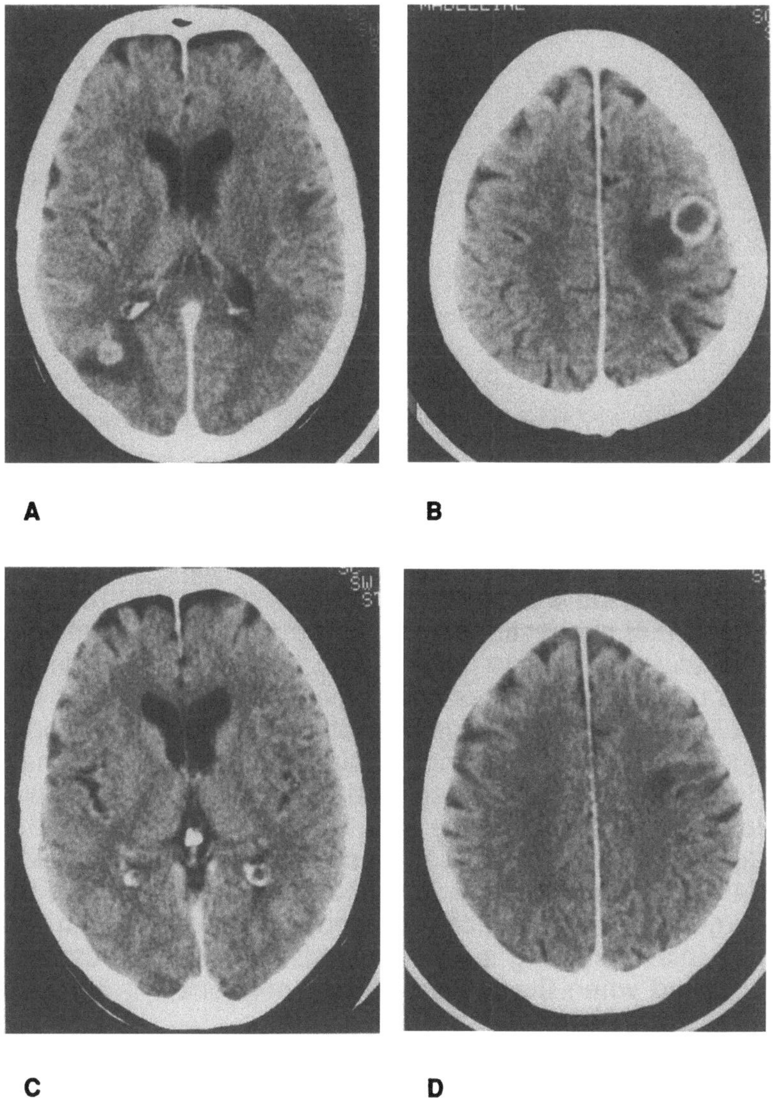

Fig. 1. A and B: Brain metastases from a primary lung cancer (squamous carcinoma). C and D: Response 1 month after RT and chemotherapy (cisplatin/5-FU)

a second chemotherapy with the same degree of effectiveness as the first one. The role of chemotherapy in the treatment of brain metastases from breast cancer deserves further evaluation. Just as for brain metastases from the lungs, Takakura, in an uncontrolled retrospective study, obtained a better median survival for patients treated with chemotherapy and radiotherapy than for patients treated with radiotherapy alone (13.2 versus 6 months).

Finally, there have been reports of remission or prolonged stabilisation (30 to 58 months) for brain metastases treated with tamoxifen [64].

Treatment of Brain Metastases from Melanomas

Brain metastases are found at autopsy in 75% of patients with melanomas. The patients' death is directly attributable to these metastases in more than half of the cases.

Preventive antiepileptic treatment is recommended.

The brain metastases respond to radiotherapy in one-third of cases [65-67], more often when they are single than when they are multiple (52% versus 30% in Katz's series) [67]. The median survival is 3 months after radiotherapy and 9 months after surgical re-

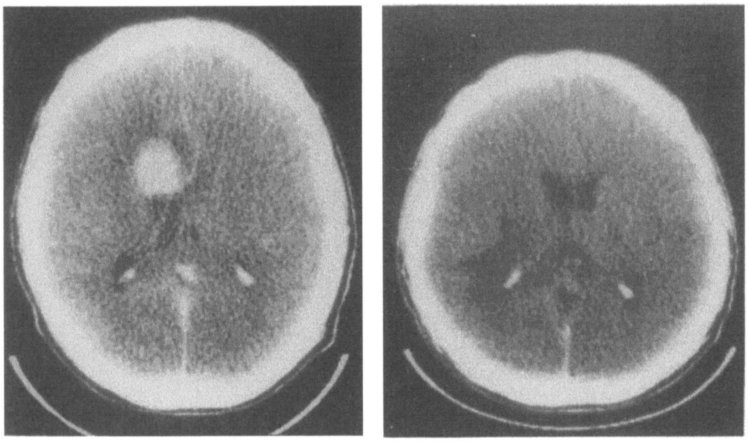

A B

Fig. 2. A: Brain metastases from melanoma. B: Response 6 months after RT

moval of a single brain metastasis. As the brain metastasis is often the cause of death, Brega [68] suggested extending the surgical indications to include patients who also have extracranial metastases and some who have multiple brain metastases. Radiotherapy after surgical removal of a single brain metastasis does not seem to affect survival but it seems to delay local recurrence and to reduce the deaths from neurological causes from 85% to 24% [8]. Radiotherapy in conjunction with surgery is therefore recommended, whenever possible. Very long survival periods may be obtained when the melanoma has only one metastatic site which is completely excised. A radiotherapy dose of 40 to 50 Gy is then recommended with fractions of 1.8 to 2 Gy in order to limit radioinduced dementia in the long term [8]. Protocols with high doses per fraction [69,70] or hyperfractionated doses [71] have not proved to be more effective than the usual protocol of 30 Gy in 10 fractions over 15 days. In a recent study, chemotherapy with fotemustine as first-line treatment gave results which were at least comparable with results from radiotherapy alone, with a response in 28% of the cases and a 26-week survival rate (Table 7).

Table 7. Treatment of brain metastases from melanoma

Series	Year	No. pts.	Treatment	Protocol	Response	Median survival (months)	1-year survival
Hilaris [89]	1963	27	RT	-	67%	4	-
Gottleib [90]	1972	41	RT	30 Gy / 2 weeks	39%	3	2%
Withers [91]	1976	100	RT	30 Gy / 1 week to 42.5 Gy / 2 wks	-	4	15%
Amer [92]	1978	16	RT	40-60 Gy / 4-6 wks	37%	4	-
Cooper [66]	1980	30	RT	20-44 Gy / 1-4 wks	35%	-	-
Carella [93]	1980	60	RT	10-40 Gy / 1-20 fr	-	2.5-3.5	-
Cairncross [2]	1980	23	RT	39 Gy / 17 days	-	2.5	0%
Katz [67]	1981	63	RT	variable	42%	3	-
Byrne [65]	1983	66	RT	39 Gy / 11 fr and 30 Gy / 6 fr	12%	2-3	-
Amer [92]	1978	4	S	-	-	22	-
Ziegler [70]	1986	13	S	-	-	10	-
Hagen [8]	1990	16	S	-	-	8.5	36%
Hagen [8]	1990	19	S+RT	24-40 Gy / fr of 2-3 Gy	-	6.5	41%
Byrne [65]	1983	9	S+RT	-	-	10	-
Jacquillat [51]	1990	39	C	Fotemustin	28%	6.5	21%

RT = radiotherapy; S = Surgery; C = chemotherapy

REFERENCES

1 Cairncross JG, Posner JB: The management of brain metastases. In: Walker (ed) Oncology of the Nervous Systems. Martinus Nijhoff, Boston 1983 pp 341-377
2 Cairncross JG, Kim JH, Posner JB: Radiation therapy for brain metastases. Ann Neurol 1980 (7):529-541
3 Takakura K, Keiji S, Shuntaro H, Asao H: Glucocorticoid therapy. In: Takakura K (ed) Metastatic Tumors of the Central Nervous System. Igaku-Shoin, Tokyo-New York 1982 pp 244-248
4 Ehrenkranz JR, Posner JB: Adrenocorticosteroid hormones. In: Weiss L, Gilbert HA, Posner JB (eds) Brain Metastases. GK Hall, Boston 1980 pp 340-363
5 Cohen N, Strauss G, Lew R, Silver D, Recht L: Should prophylactic anticonvulsivants be administered to patients with neurologicaly-diagnosed cerebral metastases? A retrospective analysis. J Clin Oncol 1988 (6):1621-1624
6 Delattre JY, Safai B, Posner JB: Erythema multiforme and Stevens-Johnson syndrome in patients receiving cranial irradiation and phenytoin. Neurology 1988 (38):194-198
7 Hoang-Xuan K, Delattre JY, Poisson M: Stevens-Johnson syndrome in a patient receiving cranial irradiation and carbamazepine. Neurology 1989 (40):1144-1145
8 Hagen NA, Cirrincione C, Thaler HT, De Angelis L: The role of radiation therapy following resection of single brain metastasis from melanoma. Neurology 1990 (40):158-160
9 Wilson CB: Brain metastases: the basis for surgical selection. Int J Radiat Oncol Biol Phys 1977 (2):169-172
10 Paillas JE, Pellet W: Brain metastases. In: Vinken PJ and Bruyn GW (eds) Handbook of Clinical Neurology. North Holland Publishing Company, Amsterdam 1975 pp 201-232
11 Tumarello D, Porfiri E, Rychlicki F, Miseria S, Cellerino R: Non small cell cancer: neuroresection of solitary intracranial metastasis followed by radio-chemotherapy. Cancer 1985 (56):2569-2572
12 Rustin GJ, Newlands ES, Begent RH et al: Weekly alternating etoposide, methotrexate and actinomycin / vincristine and cyclophosphamide chemotherapy for the treatment of CNS metastases of choriocarcinoma. J Clin Oncol 1989 (7):900-903
13 Posner JB: Surgery for metastases to the brain. N Engl J Med 1990 (322):544-545
14 White KT, Fleming TR, Laws ER: Single metastases to the brain. Mayo Clin Proc 1981 (56):424-428
15 Galicich JH, Sundaresan N, Arbit E, Passe S: Surgical treatment of single brain metastases: factors associated with survival. Cancer 1980 (45):381-386
16 Patchell RA, Tibbs PA, Walsh JW et al: A randomized trial of surgery in the treatment of single metastases to the brain. N Engl J Med 1990 (322):494-500
17 Zimm S, Wampler JL, Stablein D et al: Intracerebral metastases in solid tumor patients: natural history and results of treatment. Cancer 1981 (48):384-394
18 Gelber R, Larson M, Bolgert B, Kramer S: Equivalence of radiation schedules for the palliative treatment of brain metastases in patients with favorable prognosis. Cancer 1981 (48):1749-1753
19 Hendrickson FR: The optimum schedule for palliative radiotherapy for metastatic brain cancer. Int J Radiat Oncol Biol Phys 1981 (7):891-895
20 Kurtz JM, Gelber R, Brady L, Carella RJ, Cooper JS: The palliation of brain metastases in a favorable patient population: a randomized clinical trial by the radiation therapy oncology group. Int J Radiat Oncol Biol Phys 1981 (7):891-895
21 Young DF, Posner JB, Chu F, Nisce L: Rapid course radiation therapy of cerebral metastases: results and complications. Cancer 1974 (34):1069-1076
22 De Angelis LM, Delattre JY, Posner JB: Radiation induced dementia in patients cured of brain metastases.Neurology 1989 (39):789-796
23 Gutin PH, Phillips TL, Wara WM et al: Brachytherapy of recurrent malignant brain tumors with removable high activity iodine 125 sources. J Neurosurg 1984 (60):61-68.
24 Larson DA, Gutin PH, Leibel SA et al: Stereotaxic irradiation of brain tumors. Cancer 1990 (65):792-799
25 Roberts DW, Coughlin CT, Wong TZ et al: Interstitial hyperthermia and iridium brachytherapy in treatment of malignant glioma. J Neurosurg 1986 (64):581-587
26 Loeffler JS, Kooy HM, Wen PY et al: The treatment of recurrent brain metastases with stereotaxic radiosurgery. J Clin Oncol 1990 (8):576-582
27 Gutin PH, Wilson CB: Radiosurgery for malignant brain tumors. J Clin Oncol 1990 (8):571-573
28 Prados M, Leibel SA, Barnett C, Gutin PH: Interstitial brachytherapy for metastasis brain tumors. Cancer 1989 (63):657-660
29 Cairncross JG, Chernik NL, Kim JH, Posner JB: Sterilization of cerebral metastases by radiation therapy. Neurology 1979 (29):1195-1202
30 Hindo WA, De Trana FA, Lee MS et al: Large dose increment irradiation in treatment of cerebral metastases. Cancer 1970 (26):138-141
31 Sturm V, Kober B, Hover KH et al: Stereotaxic percutaneous single dose irradiation of brain metastases with a linear accelerator. Int J Radiat Oncol Biol Phys 1987 (13):279-282
32 Marin-Grez M, Kimmig B, Engenhart R et al: High dose percutaneous stereotaxic irradiation of solitary brain metastases using a 15 Mev linear accelerator. Int J Radiat Oncol Biol Phys 1988 (15 Suppl):230-231
33 Schwade JG, Houdek PV, Landy HJ et al: Small field stereotaxic external beam radiation therapy of intracranial lesions: fractionated treatment with a fixed halo immobilization device. Radiology 1990 (176):563-565
34 Lee JS, Umsawasdi T, Barkley HT et al: Timing of elective brain irradiation: a critical factor for brain metastases-free survival in small cell lung cancer. Int J Radiat Oncol Biol Phys 1987 (13):697-704
35 Hoskin PJ, Yarnold JR, Smith IE, Ford HT: CNS relapse despite prophylactic cranial irradiation in small cell cancer. Int J Radiat Oncol Biol Phys 1986 (12):2025-2028

36 Carmichael J, Crane JM, Bunn PA, Glatstein E, Indhe DC: Results of therapeutic cranial irradiation in small cell lung cancer. Int J Radiat Oncol Biol Phys 1988 (14):455-459
37 Baglan RJ, Marks JE: Comparison of symptomatic and prophylactic irradiation of brain metastases from oat cell carcinoma of the lung. Cancer 1981 (47):41-45
38 Lishner M, Feld R, Payne DG et al: Late neurological complications after prophylactic cranial irradiation in patients with SCLC: the Toronto experience. J Clin Oncol 1990 (8):215-221
39 Turrisi AT: Brain irradiation and systemic chemotherapy for SCLC: dangerous liaisons ? J Clin Oncol 1990: 196-199
40 Cox JD, Stanley K, Petrovitch Z, Paig G, Yesner R: Cranial irradiation in cancer of lung of all cell types. JAMA 1981 (245):469-472
41 Jacobs RH, Awan A, Bitran JD et al: Prophylactic cranial irradiation in adenocarcinoma of the lung: a possible role. Cancer 1987 (59):2016-2019
42 Ushio Y, Chernik NL, Shapiro WR, Posner JB: Metastatic tumor of the brain: developement of an experimental model. Ann Neurol 1977 (2):20-29
43 Rosner D, Nemoto T, Lane WW: Chemotherapy induces regression of brain metastases in breast carcinoma. Cancer 1986 (58):832-839
44 Shapiro WR: Chemotherapy of metastatic CNS carcinoma. In: Weiss L, Gilbert HA, Posner JB (eds) Brain Metastases. GK Hall, Boston 1980 pp 328-339
45 Cascino TC, Byrne TN, Deck MD et al: Intra-arterial BCNU in the treatment of metastatic brain tumors. J Neuro Oncol 1983 (1):211-218
46 Feun LG, Wallace S, Stewart DJ et al: Intra-carotid infusion of cisdiamine dichloroplatinium in the treatment of recurrent malignant brain tumors. Cancer 1984 (54):794-799
47 Madajewicz S, West CR, Park HC et al: Intra-arterial BCNU therapy for metastatic brain tumors. Cancer 1981 (47):653-657
48 Kristjansen PE, Hansen HH: Brain metastases from small cell lung cancer treated by combination therapy. Eur J Cancer Clin Oncol 1988 (24):545-549
49 Postmus PE, Haaxma-Reiche H, Sleijfer DT et al: High dose etoposide for brain metastases of small cell lung cancer: a phase II study. Br J Cancer 1989 (59):254-256
50 Cocconi G, Lottici R, Bisagni G et al: Combination therapy with platinium and etoposide of brain metastasis from breast carcinoma. Cancer Invest 1990 (8):327-334
51 Jacquillat C, Khayat D, Banzet P et al: Chemotherapy by fotemustine in cerebral metastasis of disseminated malignant melanoma. Cancer Chemoter Pharmacol 1990 (25):263-266
52 Robinet G, Gouva S, Clavier J, et al: Chimiothérapie par cisplatine et 5FU dans les métastases cérébrales inopérables des cancers bronchopulmonaires. Bull Cancer 1991 (78):831-837
53 Thomas P, Herkert A, Soyez F, Kleisbauer JP: Chimiothérapie des métastases cérébrales des cancers bronchiques. Rev Pneumol Clin 1990 (46):5-9
54 Takakura K, Keiji S, Shuntaro N, Asao H: Treatment. In Takakura K (ed) Metastatic Tumors of the CNS. Igaku-Shoin, Tokyo-New York 1982 pp 195-257
55 Lee JS, Murphy WK, Glisson BS et al: Primary chemotherapy of brain metastasis in small cell lung cancer. J Clin Oncol 1989 (7):916-922
56 De Angelis LM, Mandell L, Thaler HT et al: The role of postoperative radiotherapy after resection of brain metastases. Neurosurg 1989 (24):798-805
57 Patchell RA, Cirrincione C, Thaler HT, Galicich JH, Kim JH, Posner JB: Single brain metastases: surgery plus radiation or radiation alone. Neurology 1986 (36):447-453
58 Sundaresan N, Sachdev VP, Di Giacinto GV, Hughes JEO: Reoperation for brain metastases. J Clin Oncol 1988 (6):1625-1629
59 Cooper JS, Steinfeld AD, Lerch IA: Cerebral metastases: value of reirradiation in selected patients. Radiology 1990 (174):883-885
60 Kurup P, Reddy S, Hendrickson FR: Results of reirradiation for cerebral metastases. Cancer 1980 (46):2587-2589
61 Mandell L, Hilaris B, Sullivan M et al: The treatment of single cerebral metastasis from non oat cell lung carcinoma. Surgery and radiation versus radiationn therapy alone. Cancer 1986 (58):641-649
62 Kleisbauer JP, Vesco D, Orehek J et al: Treatment of brain metastases of lung cancer with high doses of etoposide (VP16-213). Cooperative study from the group français pneumo-cancérologie. Eur J Cancer Clin Oncol 1988 (24):131-135
63 Viens P, Lagrange JL, Thyss A, Ayela P, Frenay M, Schneider M: Cerebral metastases of lung cancer: excessive toxicity of high dose VP16-213. Eur J Clin Oncol 1988 (24):1905-1906
64 Pors H, von Eyben FE, Sorensen OS, Larsen M: Long term remission of multiple brain metastases with tamoxifen. J Neuro Oncol 1991 (10):173-177
65 Byrne TN, Cascino TL, Posner JB: Brain metastasis from melanoma. J Neuro Oncol 1983 (1):313-317
66 Cooper JS, Carella R: Radiotherapy of intracerebral metastatic malignant melanoma. Radiology 1980 (134):735-738
67 Katz HR: The relative effectiveness of radiation therapy in the management of melanoma metastatic to the CNS. Int J Radiat Oncol Biol Phys 1981 (7):897-906
68 Brega K, Robinson W, Winston KP, Wittenberg W: Surgical treatment of brain metastases in malignant melanoma. Cancer 1990 (66):2105-2110
69 Choi K, Withers HR, Rotman M. Intracranial metastases from melanoma: clinical features and treatment by accelerated fractionation. Cancer 1985 (56):1-9
70 Ziegler JC, Cooper JS: Brain metastases from malignant melanoma: conventional versus high dose per fraction radiotherapy. Int J radiat Oncol Biol Phys 1986 (12):1839-1842
71 Choi K, Withers HR, Rotman M: Metastatic melanoma in brain: rapid treatment or large dose fractions. Cancer 1985 (56):10-15
72 Raskin R, Weiss SR, Manning JJ et al: Survival after surgical excision of single metastatic brain tumors. Am J Roentgenol Radium Ther Nucl Med 1971 (111):323-328

73 Haar F, Paterson RH: Surgery for metastasis intracranial neoplasm. Cancer 1972 (30):1241-1245
74 Ransohoff J. Surgical management of metastatic tumors. Sem Oncol 1975 (2):21-28
75 Winston KR, Walsh JW, Fisher EG: Results of operative treatment of intracranial metastatic tumors. Cancer 1980 (45):2639-2645
76 Berry HC, Parker RG, Gerdes AJ: Irradiation of brain metastases. Acta Radiol Ther 1974 (13):535-544
77 Markesbery WR, Brooks WH, Gupta GD et al: Treatment for patients with cerebral metastases. Arch Neurol 1978 (35):754-756
78 Hildebrand J, Brihaye J, Wagenknecht L, Michel J, Kenis Y: Combination therapy with CCNU, vincristine and methotrexate in primary and metastatic brain tumors. Eur J Cancer 1975 (1):585-587
79 Twelves CJ, Souhami RL, Harper PJ et al: The response of cerebral metastases in small cell lung cancer to systemic chemotherapy. Br J Cancer 1990 (61):147-150
80 Kleisbauer JP, Guerin JC, Arnaud A, Poirier R, Vesco D: Chimiotherapie par cisplatine à forte dose dans les métastases cérébrales des cancers du poumon. Bull Cancer 1990 (77):661-665
81 Deeley TJ, Edwards JMR: Radiotherapy in the management of cerebral secondaries from bronchial carcinoma. Lancet 1968 (1):1209-1213
82 Horton J, Baxter DH, Olson KB: The management of metastases of the brain by irradiation and corticosteroids. Am J Roentgenol Radium Ther Nucl Med 1971 (3):334-335
83 Montana GS, Meacham WF, Caldwell WL: Brain irradiation for metastatic disease of lung origin. Cancer 1972 (29):1477-1480
84 Hazra T, Mullins GM, Lott S: Management of cerebral metastases from bronchogenic carcinoma. John Hopkins Med J 1972 (130):377-383
85 Gilbert H, Kagan AR, Wagner J et al: The functional results of treating brain metastases with radiation therapy. John Hopkins Med J 1972 (130):269-278
86 Nugent JL, Bunn PA, Matthews MJ et al: CNS metastases in small cell bronchohenic carcinoma: increasing frequency and changing pattern with lengthening survival. Cancer 1979 (44):1885-1893
87 Di Stefano A, Yap HY, Hortobagyi GN et al: The natural history of breast cancer patients with brain metastases. Cancer 1979 (44):1913-1918
88 Lange OF, Schee FW, Haase KD: Palliative radiochemotherapy with ifosfamide and BCNU for breast cancer patients with cerebral metastases. Cancer Chemother Pharmacol 1990 (26):78-80
89 Hilaris BS, Raben M, Calabrese M, et al: Value of radiation therapy for distant metastases from malignant melanomas. Cancer 1963 (16): 657-673
90 Gottleib JA, Frei E, Luce JK: An evaluation of the management of patients with cerebral metastases from malignant melanoma. Cancer 1972 (29):701-705
91 Withers HR, Harter D: Radiotherapy in management of malignant melanoma. In: Neoplasms of the Skin and Melanoma. Year Book Pub Co, Chicago 1976 pp 453-459
92 Amer MH, Al-Sarraf M, Baker LH, Vaitkevicius VK: Malignant melanoma and CNS metastases: incidence, diagnosis, treatment and survival. Cancer 1978 (42):660-668
93 Carella RJ, Gelber R, Hendrickson FR et al: Value of radiation therapy in the management of patients with cerebral metastases from malignant melanoma. Cancer 1980 (45):679-683

Treatment of Leptomeningeal Metastases

D. Gangji

Unité de Chimiothérapie, Hôpital Erasme, School of Medicine, Université Libre de Bruxelles, Bruxelles, Belgium

Leptomeningeal metastases are mainly encountered in children with acute lymphoblastic leukaemia (ALL) and in patients with lymphoma. Currently they are being diagnosed with increasing frequency in patients with non-haematologic malignancies such as breast and lung carcinoma, as more effective treatments are prolonging their survival. A heightened awareness of this complication may also play a role in the apparent increase of its frequency. Because of the poor outcome and the limited number of drugs available for intrathecal (IT) use, it is important to comprehend the factors that impact on treatment efficacy: mainly biology of tumour cells and drug kinetics in the leptomeningeal space.

Tumour Cell Biology in the Leptomeningeal Space

Meningeal carcinomatosis is characterised by a diffuse and widespread multifocal infiltration of the leptomeninges. Usually it will consist of several layers of cells but nodular foci may also be found. In advanced stages of the disease a deeper seated infiltration will occur with invasion of brain sulci, Virchow-Robin perivascular spaces and even brain parenchyma [1-3]. For these deeper infiltrations and the nodular lesions, drug penetration from the cerebrospinal fluid (CSF) will be limited. Nodules over 5 mm in diameter have been shown to have a poor drug penetration [4].

Little information is available on the growth kinetics of neoplastic cells in the leptomeninges. Yet this information is of paramount importance for the choice of the drug and the schedule of administration. Most agents used in the treatment of meningeal carcinomatosis, such as methotrexate (MTX) or cytosine arabinoside (Ara C), are cycle specific and are effective mainly in proliferating cells.

Prolonged exposure is therefore crucial for their efficacy [5]. Two studies have shown that leukaemic blasts have a longer S-phase and a lower labelling index in the CSF compared to peripheral blasts [6,7]. This accounts for a potential "kinetic resistance" that can be overcome if the cytotoxic concentration of the drug is maintained long enough to recruit a sufficient number of cells entering the S-phase. Such an approach was designed successfully by Bleyer et al. [8] with the Cxt regimen. This regimen allows a 72-hour exposure to cytocidal levels of MTX (1 mg q 12 hours for 3 days), whereas a single injection of 12 mg/m^2 provides this level for less than 32 hours. The Cxt regimen yields a response rate similar to that obtained with the standard 12 mg regimen given twice weekly for a total lower dose of MTX.

Drug Delivery and Kinetics in the Leptomeningeal Space

The blood-brain-barrier (BBB) is the major obstacle to adequate drug delivery into the CSF. Intrathecal (IT) administration will circumvent the BBB and achieve high drug concentrations with little systemic exposure. The concept of BBB should be further extended and linked to the "sink" effect of CSF turnover

[9]. Indeed, removal of the drug from the CSF plays also a major role in drug delivery and is mainly the result of 2 processes: a) bulk flow of entrained drug through normal absorption pathways of CSF; b) diffusion into the brain parenchyma and accross the capillaries. The latter process depends on the lipid solubility and other physicochemical characteristics of the drugs [10]. Drug administered in the CSF will not penetrate more than a few millimeters into the brain, therefore, only cells directly bathed by the CSF will be exposed to therapeutic concentrations [11].

Two routes of drug administration, one intraventricular, via the Ommaya reservoir (OR), the other intralumbar through lumbar puncture, circumvent the BBB. The OR has several advantages over the intralumbar route: a) it provides more consistent drug concentrations in the CSF, particulary at the ventricular level; b) it avoids extradural leakage, and c) it offers an easy access for repetitive administration and sequential drug assay in the CSF. However, a number of complications have been associated with its usage despite specific recommendations for management [12]. The mean percentage of complications compiled from 3 large series is 10.2%, the most frequent being staphylococcal infection, reservoir malfunctions, and other technical complications related to the reservoir [3,13,14].

For the previously mentioned reasons it is commonly considered that intraventricular treatment is superior to the intralumbar route, but no prospective study has established this superiority. Bleyer et al. [15] have shown, using the patient as his/her own control, that the duration of remission was longer after intraventricular compared to intralumbar treatment in patients with meningeal leukaemia. Other studies have reported a similar trend but they are not randomised and included only a small number of patients [3,16].

Ventriculocerebrospinal perfusion which combines the intraventricular and the intralumbar techniques is still an investigational approach. In this procedure the drug administered through an OR is removed via a cannula placed in the lumbar subarachnoid space. Using this method, Poplack et al. have reported remissions in meningeal leukaemia resistant to MTX administered through OR alone [17,18]. The concentrations of MTX achieved in this study were 1 to 2 log higher than those achieved through the OR.

Systemic administration of high doses even of drugs which poorly cross the BBB, such as MTX, may also achieve cytotoxic concentrations in the CSF. Although the major limitation is the systemic toxicity, this route of delivery provides an even distribution of the drug in the CSF [18-22].

Treatment Modalities

Chemotherapy

Methotrexate (MTX)

MTX remains the mainstay of IT chemotherapy for leukaemic and non-leukaemic meningeal diseases. MTX, a weak acid, has a low molecular weight and displays poor CSF penetration (CSF to plasma ratio: 0.03). Fifty percent is bound to albumin. MTX inhibits dehydrofolate reductase activity which results in depletion of intracellular pools of reduced folate. The presence of an excess of unbound intracellular MTX is necessary to arrest dihydrofolate reduction. The intracellular conversion of MTX into polyglutamate derivatives plays a major part in the cytotoxicity of MTX. These derivatives are retained even in the absence of extracellular MTX, and this retention is a function of the polyglutamate chain length present in the cell. MTX polyglutamates have a lower dissociation rate from the target enzyme compared to unbound MTX. In addition, they inhibit other folate requiring enzymes. The formation of MTX-polyglutamate complexes requires both an adequate drug concentration ($> 2 \times 10^{-6}$M MTX) and time of exposure (> 6 hours) [23-25].

MTX is a cell-cycle specific drug, and only cells engaged in DNA systhesis are susceptible to its action. Tumours with a low growth fraction and long cell cycle are likely to be less sensitive [26]. As for most cell-cycle specific drugs, the critical factor for MTX efficacy is the duration of exposure [27,28]. Because leukaemic cells appear to proliferate more slowly in the CSF than in the bone marrow, the duration of exposure is an essential factor in determining cell kill.

Several *in vitro* works suggest that the minimum cytocidal concentration for human leukaemic cells is between 5 x 10^{-7} and 2 x 10^{-6}M [29] and these figures have been confirmed in clinical practice. Indeed, Evans et al. [30] report an increased survival for patients with ALL treated systemically with MTX 1 g/m^2, who had 24-hour plasma levels higher than 2 x 10^{-6}M. Theoretically, in MTX-resistant meningeal leukaemia, concentrations superior to 10^{-6}M may be effective in overcoming mechanisms of resistance [23].
As mentioned previously, the pharmacokinetics of MTX differ when intralumbar, intraventricular or systemic routes of administration are used.

Intralumbar administration

The analysis of composite data from 76 children with ALL, treated by MTX 12 mg/m^2 for CNS prophylaxis, showed that the lumbar CSF concentration declines in a triphasic manner with a half-life of 4.5 and 14 hours, respectively, for the second and the third phase [31]. The same group had also shown that MTX kinetics in the CSF are dose independent, and that development of meningeal leukaemia is associated with MTX CSF levels approximately 1 to 2 log lower than those found in patients with effective prophylaxis [17,31].
Age and presence of meningeal neoplastic infiltration influence MTX levels in the CSF. If MTX dosage is based on body surface area (BSA), lumbar CSF levels are highly variable and will underdose children and overdose adults. Indeed, Bleyer [32] has shown that a constant dose of 12 mg compared to a BSA-based dosage will yield more consistent CSF concentrations. This is due to the fact that the extracellular fluid volumes of the CNS and BSA are poorly related.
The efficacy and lower incidence of neurotoxicity associated with the constant IT dose of MTX compared to a BSA-based dosage have been demonstrated by several studies. In particular, the Children's Cancer Study Group has demonstrated that a constant dose of intralumbar MTX was associated with a significantly lower rate of CNS relapse compared to a BSA-based dosage, as 6.9% versus 12.5% of children with ALL relapsed in the CNS ($p = 0.001$). The difference was particularly striking in high-risk patients (6% versus 27%, $p < 0.0002$) [33]. Consequently, the dosages proposed by Bleyer are as follows: <1 year: 6 mg, 1-2 years: 8 mg, 2-10 years: 10 mg. A flat dose of 12 mg is recommended for patients over 12 years [32-35].
Meningeal leukaemia has been associated with higher CSF levels of MTX after intralumbar administration of identical doses [17,34]. It is of note that similar findings have also been reported after intraventricular and high-dose systemic administration [35-37].
Patients displaying neurotoxic reactions after IT MTX have higher MTX levels compared to patients without toxicity [38]. Decreasing MTX dosage may reduce significantly the incidence of neurotoxicity as demonstrated by Bleyer et al. [31-35], who reported that only 5% of the patients had a neurotoxic reaction after dose reduction.
After intralumbar administration, MTX concentration in the plasma reaches a peak of 2 x 10^{-7}M after 3 hours, declines in a bi-exponential fashion with a terminal half-life of 24 hours, and falls bellow 1 x 10^{-8}M between 16 and 36 hours after drug administration [31]. This prolonged systemic exposure may require administration of leucovorin in order to protect patients from MTX toxicity.
Thus, monitoring of MTX levels in the CSF would enable the clinician to appropriately adjust MTX dosage in order to improve efficacy and reduce toxicity as no prognostic factor, with the exception of meningeal involvement, predicts abnormal levels of MTX.

Ventricular administration

In contrast to intralumbar administration, instillation of MTX via the OR results in a more consistent distribution throughout the CSF. Despite its use for over 20 years, definite guidelines for intraventricular MTX have not been set.
Shapiro et al. [39] reported high ventricular peak levels of 2 x 10^{-4}M after a 6 mg/m^2 intraventricular dose; peak levels fall in a triphasic manner with a respective half-life of 2, 4, and 8 hours. A concentration of over 10^{-7} M in both the ventricular and the lumbar CSF persisted over 48 hours.
Bleyer and Poplack [17] have administered 12 mg/m^2 MTX via the OR in 18 patients and found concentrations of 4.6 x 10^{-7}M at 24

hours and 2.7 x 10^{-7}M at 48 hours. MTX concentration was higher in the lumbar than in the ventricular CSF after 6 hours and remained 4.7-fold higher for 6 days. Ettinger et al. [40] used a 12 mg/m^2 IT dose and achieved a peak CSF concentration of 3.8 x 10^{-4}M, the concentration at 48 hours was 1 x 10^{-6}M with a terminal half-life of 7.4 hours. Thus, the dosage of 6 and 12 mg/m^2 achieved similar drug concentrations in the CSF at 24 hours and displayed comparable half-lives.

Bleyer et al. [8] devised a Cxt regimen consisting in the administration of 1 mg MTX every 12 hours for 3 days. This regimen maintains levels of MTX between 5 x 10^{-7} and 2 x 10^{-6}M for 72 hours. Compared to 12 mg/m^2 given twice a week, the fractionated schedule results in lower neurotoxicity and a smaller cumulative dose of MTX (54 mg versus 149 mg).

Recently, Strother et al. [41] have attempted to define an optimal schedule and studied doses ranging from 2 to 10 mg. They administered a median dose of 6 mg through the OR to 12 patients. The median peak concentration of MTX in the ventricular CSF was 4 x 10^{-4}M. Median concentrations at 24 and 48 hours were 4.6 x 10^{-6}M and 1.05 x 10^{-6}M, respectively. They found no correlation between the dose administered and the peak or the 24- and 48-hour CSF concentrations. There was also no correlation between the peak concentration and the subsequent concentrations. The mean terminal half-life was 8.1 hours, ranging from 3.2 to 19.8, similar to that reported by Shapiro et al. [39] and Bleyer and Poplack [17]. Again, no correlation was found between the dose and the MTX half-life. Although a very high intra- and interpatient variability was found in this study, the median 6 mg dose achieved a 10^{-6}M 24-hour CSF concentration in all but one patient and in 50% of the patients the 48-hour CSF level was above 10^{-6}M and remained above 10^{-7}M in all the patients.

The previously mentioned studies indicate that an intraventricular dose superior to 6 mg will not yield higher CSF concentrations at 24 or 48 hours nor prolong the exposure. Thus, the suggestion by Strother et al. [41], at least for patients older than 3 years, is to use an initial dose of 6 mg. This regimen, however, requires that a 24- or 48-hour CSF sample be obtained in order to adjust the dose by adding 6 mg if the concentration falls below 4 x 10^{-6}M at 24 hours or 4 mg if it falls below 1.10^{-6}M at 48 hours. Compared to the 1 mg q 12 h for 3 days schedule, this regime requires less frequent administration and will maintain the same drug levels for at least 72 hours [8]. Finally, whatever the dosage one may choose (although doses higher than 6 mg do not seem necessary), because of patient variability, presence of meningeal disease and blockage of CSF outflow, monitoring of MTX CSF levels is essential to adjust MTX dosage to ensure less neurotoxicity and better therapeutic levels.

Systemic administration

After systemic administration, MTX penetration into the CSF is poor (CSF plasma ratio: 0.03); however, with high-dose MTX therapeutic CSF levels can be achieved. The dosage, the high variability of systemic clearance, and the potential toxicity are important factors that should be taken into account in planning treatment with high-dose MTX. Dosage is, however, the most critical factor to achieve adequate levels in the CSF. Shapiro et al. [39] have compared CSF MTX distribution after a 50 mg IV bolus and a 500 mg/m^2 24-hour infusion. Negligible ventricular concentrations were achieved with the low dose whereas during the 500 mg/m^2 regimen, CSF concentrations of 0.5 x 10^{-6}M were maintained for 18 hours with plasma levels of 2 x 10^{-5}M.

Subtherapeutic concentrations of CSF MTX (< 10^{-6}M) have been measured with intermediate IV doses ranging from 500 mg to 2.5 g/m^2. Thus, after a 24-hour perfusion with 1000 mg/m^2, Evans et al. [42] have reported a mean CSF concentration of 0.27 x 10^{-6}M with a 300% range variation. In their study, CSF levels were best correlated with unbound serum MTX. Thyss et al. [43], comparing a 500 mg/m^2 to a 2500 mg/m^2 dose, also describe the high interindividual variation of serum and CSF levels. None of their patients receiving 500 mg/m^2 achieved therapeutic levels in the CSF, and only 44% of the patients treated with the higher dosage did so. Thyss et al. [43] report a correlation between

CSF and serum MTX only for the low dose but Bleyer and Poplack [17] have found a constant CSF to plasma ratio for doses ranging from 640 to 4000 mg/m^2/24 hours.
Using an even higher dose of 33.6 g/m^2, Balis et al. [19] have obtained therapeutic CSF levels of MTX: 3.6 x 10^{-6}M for 48 hours and concomitant serum concentration of 1 x 10^{-3}M, thus achieving a CSF to plasma ratio (0.03) comparable to that achieved at lower dosage. Thus, MTX serum levels may be used to predict CFS concentration of the drug.
After IV administration MTX is extensively metabolised into 7-hydroxy MTX (70H-MTX), which competes with MTX at a number of sites [44], and its levels in the blood are severalfold higher than those of MTX when using high-dose regimens [23]. Payet et al. [45] have studied the diffusion of 70H-MTX into the CSF and found that after a systemic MTX dose of 2.5 g/m^2, the levels of 70H-MTX in the CSF were nearly 100-fold lower than MTX concentrations. Evans et al. [42] did not detect 70H-MTX in the CSF in patients who received 1 g/m^2 of MTX. Because IT administration of MTX may be associated with systemic toxicity due to low but prolonged concentrations of MTX in plasma, leucovorin is used to rescue patients from MTX toxicity. Futhermore, high-dose MTX treatment requires the utilisation of leucovorin given over 1 to 2 days to counteract systemic toxicity. Leucovorin is very rapidly metabolised into an active compound, 5 methyltetrahydrofolate (5 MTHF). The latter penetrates poorly in the CSF where its concentration is 2 to 3 log lower than that of MTX administered intraventriculary [46]. Thyss et al. [47] have reported that 5 MTHF is cleared slowly from the CSF (CSF half-life is 85 hours compared to approximately 8 hours for MTX). Thus, repeated administration of leucovorin may result in high CSF levels of 5 MTHF.

Cytosine Arabinoside (Ara C)

Ara C, a pyrimidine nucleoside analogue, is phosphorylated intracellularly to its triphosphate derivative which interferes with DNA synthesis. As for MTX, duration of exposure above a threshold concentration is a major determinant for Ara C cytotoxicity [5]. Because of the rapid inactivation to arabinosyl uracil by cytidine deaminase, Ara C is usually administered by prolonged IV infusion. Ara C is presently the second most important drug for IT treatment. It is used in doses ranging from 30 to 100 mg twice weekly. The same spectrum of neurotoxicities as described for IT MTX has been reported for Ara C and the long-term toxicities do not appear to be different [48]. The half-life of Ara C in the CSF is longer that in the plasma because cytidine deaminase is present in low levels in the CNS [49]. Following an intraventricular administration of 30 mg in 7 children with ALL, Zimm et al. [50] have reported CSF peak concentrations of 2.10^{-6}M and CSF levels remaining above 10^{-6}M for 24 hours. Elimination of Ara C from the CSF is biphasic with an initial half-life of 1 hour and a terminal one of 3.4 hours, with little metabolism to the inactive compound arabinosyl uracil (Ara U). The clearance rate of Ara C from the CSF (42 ml/min) was found to be similar to the rate of CSF bulk flow (35 ml/min). Zimm et al. [50] suggest that increasing the intraventricular dose may not be necessary as comparable 24-hour drug levels would be achieved with a 30 mg or 70 mg dose and indicate that a 30 mg dose daily for 3 consecutive days will maintain a cytocidal level of 1 x 10^{-6}M for 72 hours. After intraventricular administration of 30 mg Ara C, plasma levels remain below 1 x 10^{-6}M, with no systemic toxicity [50].
Fulton et al. have studied intraventricular Ara C pharmacokinetics after a 12 mg dose in 6 patients [51]. They found a biphasic disappearance curve with a second phase half-life of 3.5 hours and CSF levels below 0.5 x 10^{-6} M at 28 hours. They also studied a 3-day regimen with 20 mg Ara C daily that produced levels above 1.5 x 10^{-6}M for 72 hours. These data suggest that a daily administration of intraventricular Ara C for 3 consecutive days may maintain concentrations above 1.10^{-6}M for more than 72 hours.
Recently, Kim et al. [52] have reported a phase I study with a slow release formulation of Ara C entrapped in multivesicular liposomes administered intraventricularly. The terminal half-life of free Ara C was increased from 3 to 11 hours. This depot form allows prolonged therapeutic drug concentrations after a single administration.
After intravenous bolus of Ara C, pharmacokinetic studies have indicated a high de-

gree of penetration into the CSF [49]. Ara C has been shown to cross the BBB as effectively at standard dose (100 mg/m^2) as at high dose (3 g/m^2). The CSF concentrations are linearly related to the dose, ranging from 347 µg/ml after 1g/m^2 to 1070 µg/ml after 3 g/m^2. The CSF concentrations range from 6 to 20% of plasma levels, and the duration of infusion does not influence the CSF concentration [53]. The use of high-dose intravenous Ara C will thus achieve cytocidal levels in the CSF and can be used for the treatment of meningeal neoplastic disease [20].

Because there is no cross-resistance between Ara C and MTX, and the combination of Ara C and MTX has been reported to be synergistic *in vitro* [54], it is current practice to use intrathecal Ara C in combination with MTX. However, in order to obtain a synergistic effect, dose and timing of administration of the two drugs should be carefully chosen to avoid antagonism between Ara C and MTX [55]. Concomitant intrathecal administration of Ara C does not modify the pharmacokinetics of MTX in the CSF [56].

Triethylenethiophosphamide (thio-TEPA)

Thio-TEPA is a polyfunctional alkylating agent mainly used in the treatment of breast and ovarian cancer. It can be administered intrathecally and is usually only used for meningeal disease refractory to MTX or Ara C or in combination with MTX and Ara C [57]. The usual intralumbar or intraventricular dosage is 10 mg once a week, yielding peak CSF concentrations ranging between 20-200 µg/ml. A higher dosage could be used but requires further investigation. Strong et al. [58] have studied plasma and CSF levels after intraventricular and intravenous administration in monkeys. After intraventricular administration, thio-TEPA levels drop very rapidly due to the clearance rate which is 9-fold faster than the CSF bulk flow. This rapid disappearance from the CSF most likely reflects a high transcapillary transport [10]. In contrast, Grochow et al. [59] measured a 4-hour CSF half-life of thio-TEPA after intraventricular administration in 13 patients and found a 0.5 ratio between ventricular and lumbar CSF. After intravenous administration to monkeys, Strong et al. [58] have shown that plasma thio-TEPA levels rapidly equilibrate with CSF, decay thereafter in a similar fashion, and result in a comparable exposure for all compartments of the CSF. After systemic administration, TEPA, a metabolite with a more potent alkylating capacity than the parent drug, is formed. Plasma Tepa levels readily equilibrate with the CSF compartment. Tepa displays a slower elimination rate from the CSF compared to thio-TEPA, resulting in a longer exposure of the CNS [58]. Furthermore, Tepa is not present in any significant amount in the CSF after intraventricular administration of thio-TEPA. Similar findings were observed by Heideman et al. [60] in one patient with a CSF to plasma ratio of 1.01 and 0.95 for Tepa and thio-TEPA, respectively. These data suggest that the standard IT administration of 10 mg once weekly may not be optimal to treat meningeal neoplasms with thio-TEPA and that novel schedules or modalities including systemic administration should be explored.

L-asparginase

L-asparginase exerts its activity by hydrolysing aspargine to aspartic acid and ammonia, thus depriving cells of this essential amino acid. Although L-asparginase has been administered intrathecally [61-63], there have been no clinical reports during the last 2 decades regarding IT administration of L-asparginase. Riccardo et al. [64] have studied L-asparginase and aspargine levels in the CSF of rhesus monkeys following intraventricular or intravenous administration. Their study shows that, although L-asparginase is cleared from the CSF faster than the bulk flow, it depletes CSF aspargine for at least 5 days.

However, a similar depletion of aspargine is observed after intravenous administration of L-asparginase. Riccardo et al. [64] followed CSF aspargine levels in 5 children with ALL and showed that aspargine depletion in the CSF occurred after systemic administration, but was not maintained over the whole 7-day period with a weekly dose of 10,000 U/m^2. Their work suggests that systemic L-asparginase may be useful in the treatment of meningeal ALL leukaemia, and indeed remissions of CNS leukaemia have been documented after systemic administration [63]. The optimal dose and schedule remain to be established.

Corticosteroids

Although corticosteroids have a lympholytic effect, and are part of the induction and maintenance treatment regimens in leukaemia and lymphomas, they are not used intrathecally to treat meningeal carcinomatosis. However, that they may have an impact on CNS disease is suggested by a randomised trial in which children with ALL who received systemic dexamethasone had the rate of meningeal leukaemia reduced by half compared to that of the prednisone-treated group [65]. A possible explanation of this result could be linked to differences in pharmacokinetics as suggested by the study by Balis et al. performed in an animal model [66]. These autors have shown that after intravenous administration the CSF to plasma ratio is higher for dexamethasone (0.15) than for prednisolone (0.08). Other factors which could also account for the higher activity of dexamethasone are its longer CSF half-life and greater proportion of unbound drug compared to prednisone. Balis et al. [66] suggest that CSF prednisolone levels achieved with standard dose are 5 to 10-fold lower than those obtained with an equipotent dose of dexamethasone. Furthermore, Pieters et al. [67] have recently demonstrated that the *in vitro* sensitivity of ALL blasts to dexamethasone is much higher compared to prednisolone than the currently assumed factor 7. With an intralumbar dose of 12 mg/m^2, it was common practice to use IT hydrocortisone for the prevention of chemical arachnoditis or acute reactions to IT chemotherapy and it resulted in a significant reduction of these side effects [68-70]. However, with improved dosage schedule and utilisation of OR, neither the need nor the efficacy of IT hydrocortisone has been demonstrated. In addition, *in vitro* data suggest that corticosteroids may interfere with the antineoplastic effect of several chemotherapeutic agents. Both cortisone and prednisolone, but not dexamethasone, have been shown to impair MTX cellular penetration [71,72]. Furthermore, adverse reactions to IT cortisone, although rare, have been reported [16]. Thus, the author does not recommend the concomitant use of IT corticoids and chemotherapeutic agents.

Diaziquone

Diaziquone (AZQ) is a highly lipid soluble alkylating agent which undergoes hepatic metabolism. It has been shown to be active against CNS tumours after systemic administration but it is associated with severe myelosuppression [73]. In humans, plasma protein binding is 79%. Following IV infusion AZQ penetrates the CSF to a significant degree both in animals [74] and in humans [75] with a CSF to plasma ratio of 0.3 .
Berg et al. [76] have reported a phase I/II trial with IT adminstration in refractory meningeal malignancies. Patients were treated intrathecally either with 1 or 2 mg bolus twice weekly or a continuous Cxt regimen using 0.5 mg q 6 hours for 3 doses. CSF levels of 6.10^{-7}M were achieved during at least 5 hours following intraventricular administration of 1 mg. Concentrations greater than 3.10^{-7}M were maintained for 18 hours after the Cxt regimen. Levels above 1.10^{-7}M have been shown to inhibit tumour growth *in vitro*.
Pharmacokinetic analysis indicates that the clearance rate from ventricular CSF is similar to CSF bulk flow (clearance: 0.37 ml/min, t 1/2: 78.6 minutes). AZQ is not metabolised in the CSF and is not detected in the plasma after IT administration. In contrast to results from animal studies [74], the ratio of ventricular to lumbar CSF of 0.1 in the study by Berg et al. [76] suggests that the drug diffuses rapidly from the CSF. Treatment was well tolerated at an 1 mg dose whereas escalation to 2 mg was limited by moderate but reversible side effects. There was neither systemic nor delayed neurotoxicity.

4 hydroxyperoxycyclophosphamide (4 HC)

Cyclophosphamide, an alkylating agent with extensive antitumour activity, is metabolised by microsomal enzymes into 4 hydroxycyclophosphamide (4 HC), its active derivative. This hepatic activation precludes the use of cyclophosphamide for regional therapy. 4 HC may be used for regional therapy as it converts spontaneously into the cytotoxic metabolite and does not require hepatic activation. Arndt et al. [77] have demonstrated in a rhesus monkey model that following IT administration, cytocidal levels of 4 HC can be achieved in the CSF. These levels cannot be

obtained after intravenous administration of cyclophosphamide because of the systemic toxicity.
Fuchs et al. [78] have reported the efficacy of 4 HC against 2 human cell lines grown in an animal model of neoplastic meningitis. In their experimental studies, there was a significant dose-dependent increase in survival and no neurotoxicity was encountered. Preliminary clinical trials are underway in patients with leptomeningeal disease.

6 mercaptopurine (6-MP)

6-MP is a purine antagonist and requires activation into its ribonucleotide derivative. It is bound to plasma protein to the extent of 30% and displays a good penetration into the CSF (CSF to plasma ratio: 0.25). 6-MP is mainly used for maintenance therapy in ALL. Covell et al. [79] have recently demonstrated the feasibility of IT administration in an animal model and have shown that most of the drug is transported out of the CSF by bulk flow, and that there is little diffusion into brain tissue. The same group has reported a phase I/II trial in children with refractory meningeal leukaemia. After IT administration of 10 mg 6-MP twice a week, 7 out 12 patients with meningeal leukaemia responded, and the toxicity was mild [80]. Considering that the half-life of 6-MP in the CSF is only 1.6 hour, Adamson et al. [80] have devised a multiple dosing schedule which maintains CSF levels of 5.9 x 10^{-6}M for 72 hours. This regimen is currently evaluated. Thus, these preliminary data indicate that 6-MP may be an active drug without significant neurotoxicity when administered intrathecally.

Radiolabelled Monoclonal Antibodies and Other Antibody Conjugates

The development of monoclonal antibodies has opened a wide field from diagnostic procedures to specific targeting of radioimmunoconjugates. Monoclonal antibody radioimmunotherapy has largely utilised I-131 and yttrium-90. These radionuclides deliver short-range energy and spare normal tissues. Leptomeningeal meningitis may consist of thin layers of cells and is particularly suitable for this type of therapeutic manoeuvres. Moseley et al. [81] have treated intrathecally 7 patients with I-131-labelled monoclonal HMFG1 antibody. Tissue distribution of the HMFG1 antigen is limited to normal and neoplastic derivatives of glandular epithelium. Clinical response was seen in 2 patients with 1 long-term survivor at 32 months. The toxicity experienced was aseptic meningitis (57%), which resolved spontaneously in all cases, bone marrow suppression (38%) and seizures. This group has also reported its experience of 15 cases treated by a single IT administration of labelled monoclonal antibody [82]. The antibody was chosen individually following demonstration of the appropriate immunoreactivity with the patient's tumour cells. CSF cytologic response was seen in 8 out 13 patients (62%), mainly in patients with medulloblastoma. They have also reported a preliminary study of patients with ALL in CNS relapse treated with IT monoclonal antibodies [83]. In a similar venue of development, Zovickian and Youle [84] have successfully tested the efficacy of a protein toxin linked to an antibody in a guinea-pig model of leptomeningeal disease. This group has recently reported a new antibody-toxin conjugate active against breast carcinoma, medulloblastoma, glioblastoma, and several solid tumour cell lines [85]. These results look very promising; monoclonal antibodies, which also provide improved methods of diagnosis, clearly offer a new avenue for regional therapy.

Cytokines

The use of biological response modifiers is a novel approach to the treatment of various neoplastic diseases. Although intraventricular administration of alpha-interferon results in a 3000-fold increase of exposure of the CNS compared to the intramuscular route [86], preliminary results with IT interferon in patients with non-neoplastic neurological diseases were not hindered by major toxicity [87]. Meyer et al. [88] have treated 9 patients suffering from leptomeningeal diseases with human leukocyte interferon at doses ranging from 3 to 9.10^6 U given 3 times a week. Although 4 of these patients cleared their CSF, 7 out of the 9 developed a vegetative state and other neurotoxic manifestations.

Experience with IT interleukin 2 (IL-2) is more limited. It has been accompanied by a considerable morbidity consisting in nausea, vomiting, fever, meningeal reactions and increased intracranial pressure. Moser et al. [89] have treated 12 patients with IT IL-2, (1.2 10^6 I.U., total dose); 9 patients responded with a survival ranging from 90 to 582 days. They also demonstrated elevated levels of tumour necrosis factor and gamma interferon and other cytokines in the CSF, following the administration of intraventricular IL-2 and report an IL-2 half-life of 4 to 8 hours [89,90].
Neuropsychiatric manifestations are protean after systemic administration of most cytokines. Therefore, close monitoring of neurotoxicity will be required in the development of IT cytokine therapy, particularly in combination with chemotherapy or radiation therapy, as toxicity may be additive.
Unless much lower doses or more appropriate drug administration schedules can be used, cytokines in the present state of development do not appear to be useful in the treatment of meningeal neoplastic involvement.

Diagnosis and Prognostic Factors

The demonstration of malignant cells in the CSF establishes unequivocally the diagnosis of meningeal carcinomatosis. False-positive results are rare, with the possible exception of patients with lymphoma because malignant lymphocytes may be difficult to differentiate from reactive cells. However, false-negative results are frequent and repeated examinations of sufficient volumes of CSF may be necessary before neoplastic cells can be identified [91]. Neoplastic cells are found less frequently in the ventricular compared to the lumbar CSF [91]. The cytospin technique has improved the yield of CSF examination [92]. The recent development of monoclonal antibodies has increased the sensitivity and the accuracy of cytologic examination [93,94]. New techniques such as flow cytometry [95], cytogenetic analysis, polymerase chain reaction and southern blot analysis for gene rearrangement will help in the detection of neoplastic cells [96].
Other non-specific but common CSF abnormalities such as low glucose and high protein levels will be found in most patients. Several tumours markers have been shown to be useful adjuncts to establish the diagnosis, e.g. beta-glucoronidase [97], lactate dehydrogenase [98], carcinoembryonic antigen (CEA) [99], beta-2-microglobuline for haematologic disorders [100], glucose phosphate isomerase [101], and tissue polypeptide antigen [102]. The sensitivity of these CSF markers varies between 30 and 70%, the lowest being for LDH; the specificity is approximatively 90%.
The lack of positive cytology will usually require other investigations. Myelography, CT scan, and gadolinium-enhanced MRI [103-105] will not only contribute to establish the diagnosis but will also help to exclude other neurological conditions, demonstrate the extent of the disease, and monitor the treatment.
Despite the widespread use of OR, drug distribution may still be inadequate due to limited patency of CSF flow in the subarachnoid space. CSF dynamic ventriculography appears to be a very useful adjunct to the management of these patients as it may indicate CSF flow abnormalities. Indeed, as many as 70% of patients with meningeal neoplastic involvement have been reported by Grossman et al. [106] to present a CSF flow blockade. Chamberlain and Corey-Bloom [107] have confirmed these results in a recent study. Fourteen out of 30 patients with meningeal carcinomatosis had compartmentalisation of CSF flow demonstrated by 111-indium ventriculography. In 6 of these patients, CSF flow blockade was not suspected on the basis of CT scan, MRI and/or clinical symptomatology. It is noteworthy that radiation therapy restored normal CSF flow in one-third of these patients. In view of these results, a 111-indium ventriculography should be obtained in all patients prior to intraventricular chemotherapy.
Definite identification of reliable prognostic factors and high-risk groups of patients is not yet established. The most important prognostic factors for treatment response and survival appear to be tumour type, progression of systemic disease and performance status [108-110]. Among non-haematologic malignancies, breast and lung cancer are the 2 tumour types responsive to IT MTX. Most CSF

parameters do not appear to be good predictors of response. One should be aware that the composition of the CSF and levels of tumour markers vary markedly between the CSF sources, i.e., ventricular or lumbar CSF [91,108]. Low glucose levels in the CSF are considered to parallel the volume of neoplastic cells and have been correlated with a poor prognosis in several series [19,108-111].
The prognostic value of high protein levels in the CSF has not been found consistently in all studies [19,108-111]. The number of cells, levels of tumour markers, delay of appearance of meningeal disease, and degree of CNS dysfunction do not influence survival. Fixed nerve lesions for over 4 weeks are less likely to improve. CSF clearance of neoplastic cells occurring within 6 weeks is associated with longer survival, as are early diagnosis and treatment. Responders have a longer survival compared to non-responders [19,108-111]. Levels of tumour markers seem to parallel the clinical response and may help in assessing the clinical activity of the meningeal carcinomatosis [112-114], but this has to be established in large and prospective studies.

Therapy

Meningeal Leukaemia

Prophylactic treatment

Prophylaxis has been considered only in acute lymphoblastic (ALL) and non-lymphoblastic leukaemia (ANLL).

Children with ALL

With improved systemic treatment, meningeal leukaemia was rapidly identified as the major obstacle to increased survival in children with ALL. Before the institution of CNS prophylactic therapy, meningeal relapse occurred in as much as 70% of the patients. A dramatic reduction of CNS ALL was reported in 1972 by Aur et al. [115] after craniospinal irradiation with 24 Gy. A year later, the same group [116] confirmed the efficacy of the craniospinal irradiation and showed that replacement of spinal radiotherapy by 5 IT injections of 12 mg MTX gave equally good results and reduced the myelotoxicity. This treatment is considered as the reference treatment yielding between 5 and 10% of CNS relapse. It is still used in high-risk patients characterised by leukocytes over 50,000 cells/mm^3, age below 1 and over 10 years, and T-cell lineage ALL [117]. Radiation therapy which plays a major role in the pathogenesis of CNS abnormalities and cognitive disorders related to CNS prophylaxis, is no longer mandatory in all children with ALL. In standard-risk patients, radiation therapy may be reduced to 18 Gy [118] or even omitted without loss of efficacy [119]. In such patients, combined IT MTX and intermediate doses of intravenous MTX may be used without radiation therapy [120]. When used alone, IT MTX must be given over the maintenance therapy period [121].
Even in high-risk groups, the need for cranial irradiation remains controversial. Thus, early results by Poplack et al. [122] indicate that high-dose MTX (33.3 g/m^2), and Ara C (1 g/m^2 x 5), alternated with IT MTX and Ara C, successfully prevent CNS relapse. Also Reaman et al. [123] reported that a similar treatment was successful in children under the age of 1 year. However, these results should be considered as preliminary.
At the time of first bone marrow recurrence, the benefit of the initial CNS prophylaxis is nullified, and the treatment must be repeated. Most of the second prophylactic protocols include IT chemotherapy using MTX alone or in combination with Ara C, and omit radiation therapy.

Adults with ALL

Overall, the outcome of adults with ALL is less favourable than that of children. In recent years, however, more effective systemic therapy has improved the survival, and consequently increased the risk of CNS leukaemia to 20-60% [117]. CNS prohylaxis using IT MTX alone or in association with cranial irradiation, or systemic high-dose MTX [124,125], has been demonstrated to substantially lower the rate of CNS relapse. Recently, however, Kantarijan et al. [126] have reported 153 adults with ALL treated with systemic vincristine, doxorubicin, dexamethasone, and cyclophosphamide omitting CNS prophylaxis.

This study indicates that in low-risk adults with ALL characterised by LDH levels below 600 IU, and a percentage of cells in S plus G2 phase inferior to 14%, CNS prophylaxis is not deemed necessary.

ANLL

In several series, the overall incidence of meningeal seedings in ANLL ranges from 10-40% [117]. The risk of developing CNS relapse is higher in myelomonocytic forms (M 4 and M 5 histologies) [127] and in patients responding to chemotherapy and thus surviving longer [117].
Based on the relatively high figures (over 20%) found in their series, Wolk et al. [128] and Stewart et al. [129] consider that CNS prophylaxis is warranted in patients with ANLL. However, Cassileth et al. [130] reviewed 2 successive ECOG series gathering 569 adults with ANLL treated without specific CNS prophylaxis, and found an overall 2.5% incidence of meningeal leukaemia. They support the view that CNS prophylaxis is unnecessary in ANLL, but advocate screening lumbar punctures during induction therapy in patients with WBC counts > 40,000/mm^3.

Overt meningeal leukaemia

The development of meningeal leukaemia is of poor prognosis because this complication is difficult to irradicate, and because most of the patients will shortly experience bone marrow relapse. In ALL intraventricular administration of MTX, consisting of 12 mg twice weekly or the less neurotoxic Cxt regimen using 1 mg q 12 hours for 3 days, yields an >90% CSF clearance [9]. IT therapy combining MTX, Ara C and hydrocortisone does not further increase the response rate [131]. Without maintenance chemotherapy, the remission will last only 2 to 4 months. Therefore, monthly IT injections of either 12 mg MTX or 20 mg Ara C or triple therapy (MTX, Ara C and hydrocortisone) must follow the induction treatment.
In ANLL, Ara C may be preferred to MTX as first-line therapy, producing an approximately 50% rate of complete CSF remissions [132,133]. However, comparative studies convincingly demonstrating the superiority of Ara C are not available. In ALL or ANLL, meningeal leukaemia refractory to MTX or Ara C, AZQ 1 mg twice weekly or 0.5 mg q 6 hours x 3, produced a 62% response rate in the study by Berg et al. [76]. In such refractory patients, 6-MP will clear the CSF in 1 out of 2 patients [80]. Not all authors use IT chemotherapy to treat overt meningeal leukaemia. Systemic high-dose MTX (33.3 g/m^2 over 24 hours) [19], or Ara C (3 g/m^2 q 12 hours over 3 to 5 days) [20] has been reported to yield an 80% response rate for MTX and 100% for Ara C, but only 5 patients were treated with the latter drug. However, despite the number of active agents, there is no documented evidence that chemotherapy alone can eradicate meningeal leukaemia [134].
Craniospinal irradiation alone also induces a 90% rate of complete remissions in overt meningeal leukaemia [117,135]. Irradiation limited to the cranium is of no value (Table 1) [156]. However, a prolonged response duration has been achieved only with relatively high doses of 24 Gy [135], which may jeopardise the intensity of systemic chemotherapy. Land et al. [136] (Table 1) have reduced the spinal dose to 14 Gy without decreasing the therapeutic efficacy. In addition, studies by Cherlow et al. [137], using intensive systemic chemotherapy with 6 Gy for spinal irradiation, and by Steinhetz et al. [138], using low-dose 6-9 Gy spinal irradiation or delaying radiation therapy (18 Gy cranial and 12 Gy spinal) up to over 1 year, indicate that these less toxic regimens may be as effective as those using higher radiation doses.
In conclusion, specific prophylaxis is mandatory in childhood ALL. In high-risk patients it consists of a combination of IT MTX (12 mg x 5) associated with cranial radiation therapy with 24 Gy; in standard-risk patients radiation therapy can be omitted providing IT MTX is either combined with an at least intermediate dose of systemic MTX or IT MTX given periodically throughout the maintenance period. In adults with ALL, CNS prophylaxis is recommended only in high-risk patients. In ANLL, CNS prophylaxis consists mainly of IT Ara C but its benefit has not been firmly established. In patients with overt meningeal leukaemia, the up-front treatment combines IT MTX (Cxt regimen) either with low-dose spinal radiation therapy or higher dose with delayed irradiation. Although no comparative data exist, high-dose systemic MTX associated with low

Table 1. Randomised trials in overt CNS leukaemia*

Reference		No. patients	Randomisation		Median Remission (months)	P-value
155	SULLIVAN			- Maintenance IT MTX	16	
	1971	47	IT MTX	- Maintenance IV BCNU	3	< 0.01
				- No maintenance	4	
68	DUTTERA	31	IT MTX + Maintenance IT MTX	- Cr 24 Gy	4	< 0.05
	1973			- no RT	> 8	
159	FRANKEL		Craniospinal 20-25 Gy		7	
	1975	66	IT MTX x 8		4	0.04
			IT MTX + Maintenance IT MTX		8	0.001
156	WILLOUGHBY	17	IT MTX	- Cr 25 Gy + spinal 10 Gy	>24	
	1976			- Cr 25 Gy	4	< 0.01
157	MURIEL	32	IT MTX/DXM	- Maintenance IT MTX/DXM	18	
	1976			- Maintenance radiocolloid	12	NS
131	SULLIVAN	65	IT + Maintenance	- IT MTX/HC/A	16	
	1977			- IT MTX/HC	12	NS
158	HUMPHREY	68	IT MTX/A/HC	- Maintenance/IT TT	15	
	1977		IT A/HC IT MTX/HC	- " "	13	NS
15	BLEYER	18	Induction + Maintenance	- Single dose	1	
	1978		Intraventricular MTX	- C x t	12	NS
136	LAND	49	IT MTX/A/HC	- Cr 24 Gy	12-24	
	1985			- Cr 24 Gy + spinal 14 Gy	24-36	< 0.02

MTX = methotrexate; A = Ara C; DXM = dexamethasone; HC = hydrocortisone; IT TT = "triple therapy" with MTX + A + HC; NS = not significant; C x t = concentration x time; CR = cranial radiation; RT = radiation therapy
* from Bleyer WA [117]

dose radiation therapy could replace IT MTX. In patients refractory to MTX several agents including Ara C, AZQ, 6-MP may induce subsequent remissions.

Lymphomas

Prophylactic treatment

CNS prophylaxis should be restricted to intermediate and high grade non-Hodgkin's lymphomas (NHL) including Burkitt's lymphoma (BL), with bulky disease, jaw involvement and/or bone marrow metastases [139-141]. Specific CNS prophylaxis consists of IT MTX. In a series of 120 patients treated sequentially on 4 different protocols at the National Cancer Institute (USA), 5 out ot 18 patients who did not receive presymptomatic IT chemotherapy relapsed in the meninges compared to only 7 of 85 patients who received the treatment [140]. For instance, in Burkitt's lymphoma Nkrumah et al. have successfully used 4 doses of 15 mg IT MTX [142]. In other forms of NHL, Anderson et al. [143], using intermediate systemic MTX doses (300 mg/m^2) during induction and maintenance, administered intrathecally 7 doses of 6.25 mg MTX. However, in therapeutic schedules using systemic high-dose MTX and/or Ara C, the benefit of specific CNS prophylaxis remains uncertain [140,143]. In the study reported by Haddy et al. [140], patients who received both IT and high-dose MTX had significantly fewer CNS recurrences compared to those treated with high-dose MTX alone.

Treatment of overt meningeal lymphoma

Treatment of overt meningeal lymphoma consists of MTX usually given through OR and may be combined with radiation therapy consisting of 24 to 40 Gy delivered to the cranium and symptomatic areas. Griffin et al. [144] treated 13 patients with lymphomatous meningitis with IT MTX alone using doses as high as 25 mg; 8 patients also received whole-brain irradiation. Seven patients, most of them treated with combined therapy, improved but all died within 20 months. Bunn et al. [145] treated 14 patients with 30 Gy radiation therapy over 3 weeks and IT MTX 12-15 mg/m^2 or Ara C 30 mg/m^2 administered twice weekly until the complete disappearance of malignant cells from the CSF, and then weekly until the neurological signs and symptoms resolved. Most of the patients also received systemic chemotherapy. In 7 patients with complete response, no subsequent death was attributed to CNS lymphoma; again, most of the patients also received systemic chemotherapy. IT MTX 12.5 mg/m^2 alone was used by Ziegler et al. in 28 patients with Burkitt's lymphoma, with a complete response in nearly all patients [146]. Five patients out of 6 with advanced non-Hodgkin's lymphoma and CNS involvement responded to high doses of systemic MTX (1-7.5 g/m^2) plus citrovorum factor. Three had a complete disappearance of the neoplastic cells in the CSF [147].

In conclusion, CNS prophylaxis using IT MTX is useful in NHL with bulky disease and/or bone marrow involvement. However, its benefit in high-risk patients is not established when high-dose MTX or Ara C are administered during induction and maintenance treatment. Overt lymphomatous meningitis can be effectively treated with a combination of IT MTX and cranial irradiation (24-40 Gy) associated with irradiation of symptomatic areas. There is no indication that response rate or survival are improved with radiation therapy delivered to the CNS. The recommended doses of MTX are similar to those used in MC originating from solid tumours (see next section).

Solid Tumour Meningeal Carcinomatosis

Prophylactic treatment

Prophylactic cranial radiation is utilised to prevent CNS metastases in patients with small cell lung carcinoma. Although it does indeed reduce the percentage of patients developing brain metastases and possibly meningeal relapse, it confers no survival advantage [148,149]. For other tumour types, there is no indication that CNS preventive therapy is warranted.

Overt disease

The prognosis of this complication is poor and most patients will die within 4 to 8 weeks from diagnosis, if untreated. Significant improvement in quality of life and survival can be achieved with an aggressive therapeutic management.

The currently used treatment modalities were not specifically developed to treat meningeal involvement from solid tumours. They derive from experience gained in the management of meningeal leukaemia in children with ALL, and have not evolved substantially over the last 20 years. The lack of an uniform approach to treatment, the variability in response criteria and tumour type make the evaluation of treatment efficacy difficult. Furthermore, in contrast to the data available for meningeal leukaemia, the number of large studies is limited, most being retrospective and only two of them are randomised. A number of questions, such as the efficacy of IT MTX compared to other drugs or drug combinations, the dose of intraventricular MTX, the superiority of OR over intralumbar administration, the need and intensity of radiation therapy, the need of maintenance therapy and lastly, the role of systemic therapy, remain unsettled.

It is standard practice to administer intraventricular MTX through OR associated with cranial irradiation and/or irradiation of symptomatic spinal areas. MTX is usually administered intraventricularly twice a week until the

CSF clears, followed by weekly and then monthly administration. Table 2, which summarises some of the largest studies performed over the last 15 years, indicates that the prognosis has not changed over time. Approximately half of the patients treated with intraventricular MTX will experience clinical stabilisation or improvement and will clear the CSF (Table 2). The highest response rates have always been observed in patients with breast cancer. It is in this category of patients that long-term survivors (>1 to 2 years) have been reported in several series [108,109, 111]. However, even the prognosis of patients with breast cancer has not changed over the last 20 years. Yap et al. [111] reported a response rate of 67% with a 24-week median survival. In a more recent study, Boogerd et al. [109] observed a 50% response rate with a 20-week median survival in breast carcinoma meningeal carcinomatosis. Although the intraventricular dose of MTX has varied from 5 to 20 mg (Table 2), there is no indication that within this range the response rate is dose related. This apparent lack of correlation between dose and response is consistent with the study by Strother et al. [41] indicating that 6 mg intraventricular MTX suffice to maintain a concentration of 1.10^{-6}M for 24 hours, and that increased dosage will not yield higher CSF concentrations at 24 or 48 hours. Furthermore, in the study by Boogerd et al. [109], where 5 mg MTX was administered to maintain a 1.10^{-6}M CSF concentration, a 50% response was achieved with a median survival of 20 weeks for responders; a result comparable to that of previous studies using higher intraventricular MTX dosage.

The only large randomised study comparing the efficacy of MTX alone to other drugs has been recently performed by Grossman et al. [110]. These authors compared in a multicentre trial 10 mg of intraventricular MTX to 10 mg thio-TEPA both given twice a week, and found no significant difference in median survival between the two arms: 15.9 versus 14.1 weeks. Because of its rapid clearance from the CSF, thio-TEPA is not considered to be an optimal drug for intraventricular usage. Therefore, the data from Grossman et al. [110] suggest that the efficacy of IT MTX in the treatment of meningeal carcinomatosis is limited. The weak effect of IT MTX is further suggested by the study of Boogerd et al. [109] where 14 patients with breast cancer meningeal carcinomatosis who did not receive IT treatment, were treated with radiation therapy and systemic chemotherapy, and had a survival comparable to that of the 44 patients treated with intraventricular MTX.

The efficacy of MTX alone has not been compared in a prospective manner to that of radiation therapy nor to radiation associated with intraventricular MTX. However, several studies do indicate that patients treated with radiation therapy alone seem to fare less well than patients treated with MTX plus radiation therapy, but the numbers studied are small [16,108].

Intrathecally administered combination chemotherapy has also been tested for the treatment of meningeal carcinomatosis by several groups. These trials are summarised in Table 2. Trump et al. [150] administered 10 mg thio-TEPA on day 1, and 10 mg MTX on day 4 to 25 patients. All patients received radiation therapy to symptomatic areas of the neuraxis, systemic dexamethazone, and most of them received systemic chemotherapy. Seventy-six percent of the patients cleared the CSF and 37% improved neurologically. The mean survival was 23 weeks. Myelosuppression was the dose-limiting factor but was considered to be related to the systemic treatment. Giannone et al. [151] treated 22 patients with MTX, Ara C and thio-TEPA (Table 2). Sixty percent of the patients had a partial clinical and CSF response but the median survival was only 10 weeks. Furthermore, this regimen was associated with an unacceptable systemic toxicity. Stewart et al. [152] have used a combination of MTX, Ara C, thio-TEPA and hydrocortisone (Table 2). Although they reported a higher response rate compared to other combination chemiotherapy trials: 100% of CSF clearing and 56% of neurological improvement, the survival was only 9 weeks. Again, myelosuppression was the most frequent toxicity. The only randomised trial comparing single drug to combined therapy is the study by Hitchins et al. [16]. Patients were randomised to receive 15 mg IT MTX or 15 mg IT MTX plus 50 mg Ara C. Most patients also received IT hydrocortisone. The response rate to MTX was higher compared to that of MTX plus Ara C (61% versus 41%, $p > 0.10$) and also higher when the OR was compared to the in-

Table 2. Trials in meningeal carcinomatosis

Reference		No. Patients		IT Chemotherapy	Response (%)	Median Survival (weeks)
3	SHAPIRO 1977	67		MTX : 6.25 mg	58	18
		Breast	15			
		Lung	7			
		Lymphoma	6			
111	YAP 1982	40		MTX : 20 mg	67	24
		Breast				
148	ROSEN 1982	24		MTX : 12 mg	63	7
		Lung				
108	WASSERSTROM 1982	90		MTX : 7 mg/m2	50 (Breast 61)	23
		Breast	46		(Lung 39)	
		Lung	23			
		Melanoma	11			
150	TRUMP 1982	25		TT : 10 mg (D1)	76 (CSF)	23
		Breast	16	MTX : 10 mg (D4)	37 (neurological PR)	
		Lung	2			
		Lymphoma	4			
151	GIANNONE 1986	22		MTX : 12 mg	60 (PR)	10
		Breast	10	Ara C : 40 mg		
		Lung	7	TT : 15 mg		
		Lymphoma	2			
152	STEWART 1987	23		MTX : 15 mg	100 (CSF)	9
		Breast	3	HC : 15 mg	56 (neurological PR)	
		Lung	7	Ara C : 75 mg		
		Lymphoma	7	TT : 7.5 mg		
16	HITCHINS 1987	44		MTX : 15 mg	61	12
		Breast	13	vs	vs	vs ($p = 0.084$)
		Lung	13	MTX : 15 mg	45	7
		Lymphoma	3	Ara C : 50 mg/m2		
153	PFEFFER 1988	98		MTX : 12.5 mg	27 (CR)	10
		Breast	33		18 (PR)	
		Lung	8			
		Lymphoma	36			
109	BOOGERD 1991	44		MTX : 5 mg	50	12
		Breast		(10^{-6}M MTX)		
110	GROSSMAN 1991	59		MTX : 10 mg	0 (neurological PR)	15.9
		Breast	28	vs		vs ($p > 0.1$, NS)
		Lung	13	TT : 10 mg		14.1
		Lymphoma	11			
154	NAKAGAWA 1992	29		MTX : 5 mg		23
		Breast	8	or	31 (CSF)	
		Lung	14	MTX : 5 mg	33 (neurological PR)	

Ara C = cytosine arabinoside; HC = hydrocortisone; MTX = methotrexate; TT = thiotepa; CR/PR = complete/partial remission. All patients received some form of radiation therapy (2500-3000 rads) (cranial or symptomatic sites). Chemotherapy was administered intraventricularly twice a week. After achieving a response, the treatment interval was gradually increased from once a week to every 8 weeks for 6 to 12 months. * Survival of all patients tralumbar route (65% versus 48%, $p > 0.10$), but none of these trends was statistically significant. Survival was better on the MTX arm but not significantly so. Furthermore, the response rate for patients who received concomitant CNS radiation therapy was much higher compared to non-irradiated patients (73% versus 35%, $p < 0.05$), and their survival was longer (17.5 versus 8 weeks). Neither this randomised trial nor those mentioned above demonstrate any significant advantage for the combination chemotherapy. However, the study by Trump et al. [150] using MTX and thio-TEPA, reports one of the longest survival durations over the last 10 years (Table 2). Their treatment regimen differs from others by the fact that drugs were not administered concomitantly. This difference may be an important factor.

Meningeal carcinomatosis relapsing after MTX administration may respond to a second IT MTX treatment; however, the response duration is even shorter compared to the first one. On the other hand, meningeal carcinomatosis resistant to MTX may respond to IT Ara C or thio-TEPA. The latter should be preferred due to the greater sensitivity of solid tumours to alkylating agents compared to Ara C.

In conclusion, although the treatment is palliative, most patients will benefit from it as it may improve quality of life and possibly survival if the underlying disease can be controlled. The standard treatment of meningeal carcinomatosis complicating solid tumours combines IT MTX and 25 to 30 Gy radiation therapy delivered to the cranium and spinal symptomatic areas. A 6 mg dose of IT MTX is administered twice weekly until the CSF clears; usually the response is anticipated within 6 weeks. Thereafter 6 mg IT MTX is given weekly for 4 to 8 weeks followed by monthly treatment. At present, no combination chemotherapy appears to be superior to IT MTX alone; however, other agents such as thio-TEPA are potentially useful in meningeal metastases resistant to MTX.

Acknowledgment

The author gratefully acknowledges the support and helpful suggestions provided by Dr. J. Hildebrand.

REFERENCES

1 Price RA, Jamieson PA: The central nervous system in childhood leukemia. The arachnoid. Cancer 1973 (31):520-533
2 Olson HE, Chernik NL, Posner JB: Infiltration of the leptomeninges by systemic cancer. A clinical and pathologic study. Arch Neurol 1974 (30):122-137
3 Shapiro WR, Posner JB, Ushio Y, Chernik NL, Young DF: Treatment of meningeal neoplasms. Cancer Treat Rep 1977 (61):733-743
4 Flessner MF, Fentermacher JD, Dedrick RL, Blasberg RG: A distributed model of peritoneal-plasma transport tissue concentration gradients. Am J Physiol 1985 (248):425-435
5 Bruce WR, Meeker BE, Powers WE, Valeriote FA: Comparison of the dose and time survival curves for normal hematopoietic and lymphoma colony-forming cells exposed to vinblastine, vincristine, arabinosyl cytosine and amethopterin. JNCI 1966 (37):233-245
6 Kuo A, Yataganas X, Galicich JH, Fried J, Clarkson B: Proliferative kinetics of central nervous system leukemia. Cancer 1975 (36):232-238
7 Tsuchiya J, Moteki M, Shimano S: Proliferative kinetics of leukemic cells in meningeal leukemia. Cancer 1978 (42):1255-1262
8 Bleyer WA, Poplack DG, Simon RH: Concentration x time methotrexte via a subcutaneous reservoir: a less toxic regimen for intraventricular chemotherapy of central nervous system neoplasms. Blood 1978 (51):835-842
9 Collins JM, Dedrick RL: Distributed model for drug delivery. Am J Physiol 1983 (245):R303-R310
10 Blasberg R, Patlack CS, Fenstermacher JD: Intrathecal chemotherapy: brain tissues profiles after ventriculoperfusion. J Pharm Exp Ther 1975 (195):73-83
11 Blasberg R, Patlack CS, Shapiro WR: Distribution of methotrexate in the cerebrospinal fluid and brain after intraventricular administration. Cancer Treat Rep 1977 (61):633-641
12 Bleyer WA, Pizzo PA, Spence AM et al: The Ommaya reservoir: newly recognized complications and recommandations for insertion and use. Cancer 1978 (41):2431-2437
13 Obens EAMT, Leavens ME, Beal JW, Lee YY: Ommaya reservoirs in 387 cancer patients: a 15 year experience. Neurology 1985 (35):1274-1278
14 Lishner M, Perrin RG, Feld R, Messner HA, Tuffnell PC, Elhakim T, Matlow A, Curtis JF: Complications associated with Ommaya reservoirs in patients with cancer. Arch Int Med 1990 (150):173-176
15 Bleyer AW, Poplack DG: Intraventricular versus intralumbar methotrexate for central nervous system leukemia. Med Ped Oncol 1979 (6):207-213
16 Hitchins RN, Bell DR, Woods RL, Levi JA: A prospective randomized trial of single-agent versus combination chemotherapy in meningeal carcinomatosis. J Clin Oncol 1987 (5):1655-1662
17 Bleyer WA, Poplack DG: Clinical studies on the CNS pharmacology of methotrexate. In: Pinedo HM (ed) Clinical Pharmacology of Antineoplastic Drugs. Elsevier Biomedical Press, Amsterdam 1978 pp 115-135
18 Poplack DG, Bleyer WA, Pizzo PA: Experimental approaches to the treatment of CNS leukemia. Am J Ped Hematol Oncol 1979 (1):141-149
19 Balis FM, Savitch JL, Bleyer WA, Reaman GH, Poplack DG: Remission induction of meningeal leukemia with high-dose intravenous methotrexate. J Clin Oncol 1985 (3/2):485-489
20 Frick J, Ritch PS, Hansen RM, Anderson T: Successful treatment of meningeal leukemia using systemic high-dose cytosine arabinoside. J Clin Oncol 1984 (2):365-368
21 Postmus PE, Hocthuis JJM, Haaxma-Reiche H: Penetration of VP16-213 into CSF after high-dose intravenous administration. J Clin Oncol 1984 (2):215-220
22 Postmus PE, Haaxma-Reiche H, Berendsen HH, Sleijfer DT: High-dose etoposide for meningeal carcinomatosis in patients with small cell lung cancer. Eur J Clin Oncol 1989 (25/2):377-378
23 Jolivet J, Cowan KH, Curt GA, Clendenin NJ, Chabner BA: The pharmacology and clinical use of methotrexate. N Engl J Med 1983 (3):1094-1104
24 Chabner BA, Allegra CJ, Curt GA, Clendeninn NJ, Baram J, Koizumi S: Polyglutamation of methotrexate. J Clin Investig 1985 (76):907-912
25 McGuire JJ, Mini E, Hsies P, Bertino JR: Role of methotrexate polyglutamates in methotrexate and sequential methotrexate 5-fluorouracil mediated cell kill. Cancer Res.1985 (45): 6395-6400
26 Johnson LF, Fhurman CL, Abelson HT: Resistance of resting mouse fibroblasts (3 TG) to methotrexate cytotoxicity. Cancer Res 1978 (38):2408-2412
27 Keefe A, Capizzi RL, Rudnick SA: Methotrexate and cytotoxicity for L5178Y/ASN lymphoblasts: relationship of dose and duration of exposure to tumor cell viability. Cancer Res 1982 (42):1641-1645
28 Gangji D, Ducore J, Poplack D, Kohn K, Glaubiger D: Concentration and time dependence of methotrexate cytoxicity in mouse L1210 leukemia cells and human Burkitt's lymphoma cells. Clin Res 1980 (28):525
29 Chabner BA and Younger RC: Threshold methotrexate concentration for in vivo inhibition of DNA synthesis in normal and tumorous target tissue. J Clin Invest 1973 (52):1804-1811
30 Evans WE, Crom WR, Abromowitch M, Dodge R, Look T, Bowman WP, George SL, Pui CH: Clinical pharmacodynamics of high-dose methotrexate in acute lymphocytic leukemia. Identification of a relation between concentration and effect. N Engl J Med 1986 (314):471-477
31 Bleyer WA, Dedrick RL: Clinical pharmacology of intrathecal methotrexate I. Pharmacokinetics in non-toxic patients after lumbar injection. Cancer Treat Rep 1977 (61):1419-1425
32 Bleyer WA, Dedrick RL: Clinical pharmacology of intrathecal methotrexate II. An improved dosage schedule derived from age-related pharmacokinetics. Cancer Treat Rep 1977 (61):1419-1421
33 Bleyer WA, Coccia PF, Sather HN, Level C, Lukens J, Neibrugge DJ, Siegels S, Littman PS, Leikin SL,

Miller DR, Chard RL, Hammond GD: Reduction in the CNS leukemia with a pharmacokinetically derived intrathecal methotrexate dosage regimen. J Clin Oncol 1983 (1):317-325
34 Bleyer AW: Clinical pharmacology of intrathecal methotrexate; an improved dosage regimen derived from age related pharmacokinetics. Cancer Treat Rep 1977 (61):1419-1425
35 Bleyer WA, Savitch JL, Holcenberg JS: An improved regimen for intrathecal chemotherapy. Clin Pharmacol Exp Ther 1976 (19): 103-104
36 Dufner PK, Cohen ME, Brecher ML, Berer D, Parthasarathy KL, Bakshi S, Ettinger LF, Freeman A: CT abnormalities and altered methotrexate clearance in children with CNS leukemia. Neurology 1984 (34):229-233
37 Morse M, Savitch J, Balis F, Miser J, Feusner J, Reaman G, Poplack DG, Bleyer AW: Altered central nervous system pharmacology of methrotexate in childhood leukemia: Another sign of meningeal relapse. J Clin Oncol 1985 (3):19-24
38 Bleyer WA, Drake JC, Chabner BA: Neurotoxicity and elevated CSF MTX concentrations in meningeal leukemia. N Engl J Med 1973 (289):770-773
39 Shapiro WR, Young DF, Metha BM: Methotrexate: distribution in CSF after intravenous, ventricular and lumbar injections. N Engl J Med 1975 (293):161-166
40 Ettinger LJ, Chervinsky DS, Freeman AI: Pharmacokinetics of methotrexale following intravenous and intraventricular administration in acute lymphocytic leukemia and non-Hodgkin's lymphoma. Cancer 1982 (50):1676-1682
41 Strother DR, Glynn-Barnhart A, Kovnar E, Gregory RE, Murphy: Variability in the disposition of intraventricular methotrexate: a proposal for matinal dosing. J Clin Oncol 1989 7:1741-1747
42 Evans WE, Hutson PR, Stewart CF, Cairness DA, Powman P, Rivera G, Crom WR: Methotrexate CSF and serum concentrations after intermediate-dose infusion. Clin Pharmacol Ther 1983 (33):301-307
43 Thyss A, Milano G, Deville A, Manassero J, Renee N, Schneider M: Effect of dose and repeat intravenous 24 hr infusions of methotrexate on cerebrospinal fluid availability in children with hematological malignancies. Eur J Cancer Clin Oncol 1987 (23):813-817
44 Fabre I, Fabre G, Cano JP: 7 hydroxymethotrexate cytotoxicity and selectivity in a human Burkitt's lymphoma cell line versus granulocytic progenitor cells: rescue by folinic acid and nucleosides. Cancer Clin Oncol 1986 (22):1247-1254
45 Payet B, Tubiana N, Lejeune C, Guerin B, Cano JP, Carcassone Y: High-dose methotrexate: methotrexate and 7-hydroxymethotrexate diffusion in CSF. Int J Cancer 1988 (42):135-136
46 Mehta BM, Glass JP, Shapiro WR: Serum and cerebrospinal fluid distribution of 5 methyltetra-lydropolate after intravenous calcium leucovorin and intra Ommaya methotrexate administration in patients with meningeal carcinomatosis. Cancer Res 1983 (43):435-438
47 Thyss A, Milano G, Etienne MC, Paquis P, Roche JL, Grelier P, Schneider M: Evidence of CSF accumulation of 5 methyltetrahydrofolate during repeated course of methotrexate plus folimic acid rescue. Br J Cancer 1989 (59):627-630
48 Peylan Ramu N, Poplack DG, Pizzo PA, Adonarto BT, Di Chiro A: Abnormal computed tomography of the brain in asymptomatic children with acute lymphoblastic leukemia following central nervous system prophylaxis. N Engl J Med 1978 (299):815-181
49 Ho DHW: Potential advances in the clinical use of arabinosyl cytosine. Cancer Treat Rep 1977 (61):712-722
50 Zimm S, Collins JM, Miser J, Chatterji D, Poplack DG: Cytosine arabinoside cerebrospinal fluid kinetics. Clin Pharmacol Ther 1984 (35):826-830
51 Fulton DS, Levin VL, Gutin PH: Intrathecal cytosine arabinoside for the treatment of meningeal metastases from malignant brain tumors and systemic tumors. Cancer Chemother Pharmacol 1982 (8):285-291
52 Kim S, Chatelut E, Khatibis S, Kim J, Howell SB, Chamberlain MC: Leptomeningeal metastasis: pharmacokinetics of cytosine arabinoside (Ara C) encapsulated in depot form administered intraventricularly. Proceed Am Soc Clin Oncol 1982 (411): 148
53 Slevin ML, Piall EM, Aherne GW: Effect of dose and schedule on pharmacokinetics of high-dose cytosine arabinoside in plasma and cerebrospinal fluid. J Clin Oncol 1983 (1):546-551
54 Avery TL, Roberts D: Dose related synergism of cytosine arabinoside and methotrexate against murine leukemia L1210. Eur J Cancer 1974: 425-429
55 Cadman E and Eiferman F: Mechanism of synergistic cell killing when methotrexate precedes cytosine arabinoside. J Clin Invest 1979 (64):788-797
56 Gangji D, Cohen L, Bleyer WA, Vigerski R, Glaubiger D, Poplack DG: Methotrexate CNS pharmacokinetics in combination chemotherapy in CNS complications of malignant disease. In: Whitehouse JMA Kay HEM (eds) CNS Complications of Malignant Disease. MacMillan Press, London1979 pp 407-412
57 Gutin DH, Levi JA, Wiernik PH, Walker MD: Treatment of malignant disease with intrathecal thio-Tepa. A phase II study. Cancer Treat Rep 1977 (61):885-887
58 Strong JM, Collins JM, Lesther C, Poplack DG: Pharmacokinetics of intraventricular and intravenous N'-N"-N"-triethylenethiophosphoramide (thio-TEPA) in rhesus monkeys and humans. Cancer Res 1986 (46):6101-6104
59 Grochow LB, Grossman S, Garret S, Murray K, Trump D, Colvin M: Pharmacokinetics of intraventricular thio-Tepa with meningeal carcinomatosis. Proc Am Soc Clin Oncol 1982 (1):19
60 Heideman R, Cole DE, Balis F, Sato J, Reaman GH, Packer RJ, Singher LJ, Ettinger LJ, Gillespie A, Sam J, Poplack DG: Phase I and pharmacokinetic evaluation of thio-Tepa in the cerebrospinal fluid and plasma of pediatric patients: evidence for dose-dependent plasma clearance of thio-Tepa. Cancer Res 1989 (49):736-741

61 Tallal L, Tan C, Oettgen H, Wallner N, McCarthy N, Helson L, Burchenal J, Karnofsky D, Murphay ML: E. coli L-asparaginase in the treatment of leukemia and solid tumors in 131 children. Cancer 1970 (25):244-252

62 Tan C, Oettgen H: Clinical experience with L-Asparginase administered intrathecally. Proc Am Assoc Cancer Res 1969 (10):92

63 Schwartz M, Lash ED, Oettgen HF, Tomato F: L-Asparginase activity in plasma and other biological fluids. Cancer 1970 (25):244-252

64 Riccardo R, Hollenberg JS, Glaubiger DL, Wood JH, Poplack DG: L-Asparginase pharmacokinetics and aspargine levels in cerebrospinal fluid of Rhesus monkeys and humans. Cancer Res 1981 (41):4554-4558

65 Jones B, Shuster JJ, Holland JF: Lower incidence of meningeal leukemia when dexamethasone is subsituted for prednisone in the treatment of acute lymphocytic leukemia: a late follow-up. Proc Am Soc Clin Oncol 1984 (3):18

66 Balis FM, Lester CM, Chrousos GP, Heideman RL, Poplack DG: Differences in CSF penetration of corticosteroids: possible relationship to the prevention of meningeal leukemia. J Clin Oncol 1987 (5):202-207

67 Pieters R, Kaspers GJL, Wering ER, Hahlen K, Veerman: Dexamethasone is much more potent than prednisolone in the assumed equivalent doses in chilhood leukemia. Proc Am Soc Clin Oncol 1992 (283)

68 Duttera MJ, Bleyer WA, Pomeroy TC, Leventhal CM, Levental BG: Irradiation, methotrexate toxicity, and the treatment of meningeal leukemia. Lancet 1973 (2/7831):703-707

69 Fujimoto T, Goya G, Makagawa K, Yamashita J, Ito M, Asano K, Furusho F: Comparison of high dose infusion of methotrexate (MTX) vs sequential-complementary method for maintenance of remission in acute childhood leukemia. A comparative study. Proc 11th Ann Meeting Am Soc Clin Oncol 1975 (16):65

70 Fujimoto T, Goya N, Nakagawa K, Yamashita F, Fuji Y, Asano K, Furusho K: Chemotherapy of acute chilhood leukemia . I. Comparison of high dose infusion of MTX vs sequential-complementary method for maintenance of remission. Jpn J Clin Hematol 1974 (15):1106-1113

71 Bender RA, Bleyer WA, Frisby SA, Olivierio VT: Alteration of methotrexate uptake in human leukemia cells by other agents. Cancer Res 1975 (35):1305-1308

72 Zager RF, Frisby SA, Oliveiro VT: The effects of antibiotics and cancer chemotherapy agents on the cellular transport and antitumor activity of MTX on L1210 murine leukemia. Cancer Res 1973 (33):1670-1675

73 Schilsky R, Kelley J, Ihde D: Phase I trial and pharmacokinetic of azinidinylbenzoquinone in humans. Cancer Res 1982 (42):1582-1586

74 Zimm S, Collins J, Curt GA, O'Neill D, Poplack DG: Cerebrospinal fluid pharmacokinetics of intraventricular and intravenous azinidinylbenzo-quinone. Cancer Res 1984 (44): 1698-1701

75 Bachur NR, Collins JM, Kelley JA, Van Echo DA, Kaplan RS, Whitacre: Diaziquone 2,5 diariziridinyl-3-6 biscarbrethoxyamino 1-4 benzoquinone, plasma and cerebrospinal kinetics. Clin Pharm Ther 1982 (31):650-655

76 Berg SL, Balis FM, Zimm S, Murphy RF, Holcenberg J, Sato J, Reaman G, Steinherz P, Gillespie A, Doherty R, Poplack DG: Phase I/II trial and pharmacokinetics of intrathecal diaziquine in refractory meningeal malignancies. J Clin Oncol 1992 (10):143-149

77 Arndt CA, Colvin OM, Balis FM, Lester CM, Johnson G, Poplack DG: Intrathecal administration of 4-hydroxyperoxycylophosphamide in rhesus monkeys. Cancer Res 1987 (47/22):5932-5934

78 Fuchs HE, Archer GE, Colvin OM, Bigner SH, Schuster JM, Fuller GN, Mulbaier LH, Schold SC Jr, Friedman HS, Bigner DD: Activity of intrathecal 4-hydroxyperoxycyclophosphamide in a nude rat model of human neoplastic meningitis. Cancer Res 1990 (50):1254-1259

79 Covell D, Narang PK, Poplack DG: Kinetics model for disposition of 6 mercaptopurine in monkey plasma and cerebrospinal fluid. Am J Physiol 1985 (248):R147-R156

80 Adamson PC, Arndt CA, Balis FM, Tartaglia RL, Gillespie AF, Murphy RF, Holcenberg JS, Poplack DG: Intrathecal mercaptopurine 6MP: phase I/II trial and CSF pharmacokinetic study in children with refractory meningeal leukemia. Proc Am Soc Clin Oncol 1989 (8):213

81 Moseley RP, Benjamin JC, Ashpole RD, Sullivan NM, Bullimore JA, Coakham HB, Kem shead JT: Carcinomatous meningitis: antibody guided therapy with I-131 HMFG1. J Neurol Neurosurg Psych 1991 (54):260-265

82 Moseley RP, Davies AG, Richardson RB, Zalutsk Y, Carell S, Fabre J, Slack N, Bullimore J, Pizer B, Papanastassiou V, Kemshead JT, Coakam HB, Lashford LS: Intrathecal administration of 134 I radiolabelled monoclonal antibody as a treatment for neoplastic meningitis. Br J Cancer 1990 (62):657-692

83 Pizer BL, Papanastassiou V, Hannock J, Cassano W, Coakham H, Kemstead JT: A pilot study of MoAb targeted radiotherapy in the treatment of central nervous system leukemia in children. Br J Haematol 1991 (77):466-472

84 Zovickian J, Youle RJ: Efficacy of IT immunotoxin therapy in an animal model of leptomeningeal neoplasia. J Neurosurg 1988 (68):767-774

85 Johnson VG, Wrobel C, Wison D, Zovickian J, Greenfield L, Oldfield EH, Youle R: Improved tumor specific immunotoxins in the treatment of CNS and leptomeningeal neoplasia. J Neurosurg 1989 (70):240-248

86 Collins JM, Riccard R, Trown P, O'Neill, Poplack DG: Plasma and cerebrospinal fluid pharmacokinetics of recombinant interferon alpha in monkeys. Comparison of intravenous, intramuscular and intraventricular delivery. Cancer Drug Deliv 1985 (2):247-253

87 Kuroki S, Tsutui T, Yoshioka: The effect of intraventricular interferon on subacute sclerosing panencephalitis. Brain Dev 1989 (11):65-69

88 Meyers CA, Obens EAMT, Scheibel RS, Moser RP: Neurotoxicity of intraventricularly administered alpha interferon for leptomeningeal disease. Cancer 1991 (68):88-92
89 Moser RP, Bruner JM, Grimm EA: Biologic therapy for brain tumors. Cancer Bull 1991 (43):117-126
90 List J, Moser RP, Loudon WG, Blacklock JB, Grimm EA: Tumor necrosis factor, interleukin 1, interleukin 6, gamma interferon and soluble interleukin 2 receptor (Mr 55000 protein). Cancer Res 1991 (6):1123-1128
91 Glass JP, Melamed N, Chernik NL, Posner JB: Malignant cells in cerebrospinal fluid: the meaning of a positive CSF cytology. Neurology 1979 (29):1369-1375
92 Choi HSH, Anderson PJ: Diagnostic cytology of cerebrospinal fluid by the cytocentrifuge method. Am J Clin Path 1979 (72):931-943
93 Moseley RP, Oge K, Shafqats S, Moseley CM, Sullivan NM, Bradley RA, Burchell J, Taylor-Papadimitriou and Coakham HB: HMFGI Antigen: a new marker for carcinomatous meningitis. Int J Cancer 1989 (44):440-444
94 Hovestadt A, Henzen-Logmans SC, Vecht CJ: Immunohistochemical analysis of the CSF for carcinomatous and lymphomatous leptomeningitis. Br J Cancer 1990 (62):653-654
95 Cibas ES, Malkin MM, Posner JB, Melamed MR: Detection of DNA abnormalities by flow cytometry in cells from cerebrospinal fluid. AmJ Clin Pathol 1987 (88):570-577
96 Lange BJ, Rovera G: Detection of minimal residual leukemia in acute lymphoblastic leukemia. Hem Oncol Clin North America 1991 (4):845-995
97 Tallmon RD, Kimbrough SM, O'Brien JF, Goellner JR, Yanagihara T: Assay for beta-glucuronidase in cerebrospinal fluid: usefulness for the detection of neoplastic meningitis. Mayo Clin Proc 1985 (60):293-298
98 Van Zanten AP, Twijnstra A, Hart AAM, Ongerbroer de Visser BW: Cerebrospinal fluid lactate dehydrogenase activities in patients with central nervous system metastases. Clin Chim Acta 1986 (161): 259-268
99 Yap BS, Yap HY, Fritsche H, Blumenschein G, Bodey JP: CSF carcinoembryonic antigen in meningeal carcinomatosis from breast cancer. J Amer Med Ass 1980 (244):600-601
100 Twijnstra A, Van Zanten AP, Nooyen WJ, Hart AAM, Ongerbroer de Visser BW: Cerebrospinal fluid beta-2-microglobulin: a study in controls and patients with metastatic and non-metastatic neurological disease. Eur J Cancer Clin Oncol 1986 (22):387-392
101 Newton HB, Fleisher M, Schwartz MK, Malkin MG: Glucosephosphate isomerase as a CSF marker for leptomeningeal metastasis. Neurology 1991 (41):395-398
102 Bach F, Soletormos G, Dombernowsky P: Tissue polypeptide antigen activity in cerebrospinal fluid: a marker of central nervous system metastases of breast cancer. JNCI 1991 (83):779-784
103 Rodesch G, Van Bogaert, Mavroudakis N, Parizel PM, Martin JJ, Segebarth C, Van Vyve M, Baleriaux D, Hildebrand J: Neuroradiologic findings in leptomeningeal carcinomatosis: the value interest of gadolinium-enhanced MRI. Neuroradiology 1990 (32):26-32
104 Youssem DM, Patrone PM, Grossman RI: Leptomeningeal metastases: MR evaluation. J Comput Assist Tomogr 1990 (14):255-261
105 Phillips ME, Ryals TJ, Kambhu SA, Yuh WTC: Neoplastic vs inflammatory meningeal enhancement with Gd-DTPA. J Comput Assist Tomogr 1990 (14):536-541
106 Grossman SA, Trump DL, Chen DCP, Thompson GPA, Camargo EE: Cerebrospinal fluid flow abnormalities in patients with neoplastic meningitis. An evaluation using "indium-DTPA ventriculography". Am J Med 1982 (73):641-647
107 Chamberlain MC and Corey-Bloom J: Leptomeningeal metastases: indium-DTPA CSF flow studies. Neurology 1991 (41):1765-1769
108 Wasserom WR, Glass JP, Posner JP: Diagnosis and treatment of leptomeningeal metastases from solid tumors. Experience with 90 patients. Cancer 1982 (49):759-772
109 Boogerd W, Hart AA, Van der Sande JJ, Engelsman E: Meningeal carcinomatosis in breast cancer. Cancer 1991 (67):1685-1695
110 Grossman SA, Ruckdeschel JC, Moynihant Finkelstein D, Ettinger D, Mahoney E, Trump D: Randomized prospective comparison of intraventricular methotrexate and thio-tepa for neoplastic meningitis. Proc Am Soc Clin Oncol 1991 (10):127
111 Yap HY, Yap BS, Rasmussen S, Levens ME, Hortobagyi GN, Blumenschein GR: Treatment for meningeal carcinomatosis in breast cancer. Cancer 1983 (49):219-222
112 Twijnstra A, Ongerboer de Visser BW, Van Zanten AP, Hart AAM, Nooyen WJ: Serial lumbar and ventricular cerebrospinal fluid biochemical marker measurements in patients with leptomeningeal metastases from solid and hematological tumors. J Neuro Oncol 1989 (7):57-63
113 Schold SC, Wasserstrom WR, Fleischer M, Schwartz MK, Posner JB: Cerebrospinal fluid biochemical markers of central nervous system metastases. Ann Neurol 1980 (8):597-604
114 Van Zanten AP, Twijnstra A, Ongerboer de Visser BW, van Heerde P, Hart HAM, Nooyen WJ: Cerebrospinal fluid tumor markers in patients treated for meningeal malignancy. J Neurol Neurosurg Psych 1991 (54):119-123
115 Aur RJA, Simone JV, Hustu HO, Verzosa MS: A comparative study of central nervous system irradiation and intensive chemotherapy early in remission of chilhood lymphocytic leukemia. Cancer 1972 (29):381-391
116 Aur RJA, Hustu HO, Verzosa MS, Wood A, Simone JV: Comparison of two methods of preventing central nervous system leukemia. Blood 1973 (42):349-357
117 Bleyer WA: Central nervous system leukemia. Ped Clinics of North America 1988:789-814
118 Nesbit NE, D'Angio GJ, Sather HN, Robison LL, Ortega J, Donaldson M, Hammond GD: Effects of isolated CNS leukemia on bone marrow remission and survival in childhood acute lymphoblastic

leukemia: a report for the Children's Cancer Study Group. Lancet 1981 (i):1386-1389

119 Komp DM, Fernandez CH, Falleta JM: CNS prophylaxis in acute lymphoblastic leukemia: a comparison of two methods. Cancer 1982 (50):1031-1036

120 Abromowitch M, Ochs J, Piu CH: Efficacy of high-dose methotrexate in childhood acute lymphocytic leukemia: analysis by contemporary risk. Blood 1988 (74):866-869

121 Sullivan MP, Chen TM, Dyment PG, Hvizdala E, Steuber CP: Equivalence of intrathecal chemotherapy and radiotherapy as central nervous system prophylaxis in children with acute lymphocytic leukemia: a pediatric oncology group study. Blood 1982 (60):948-959

122 Poplack DG, Reaman GH, Bleyer WA, Feusner J, Odom S, Steinberg S, Sather H, Hammond D: Successful prevention of CNS leukemia without cranial radiation in children with high risk acute lymphoblastic leukemia: a preliminary report. Proc Am Soc Clin Oncol 1989 (8):213

123 Reaman GH, Poplack DG, Wesley R, Bleyer WA, Wiser J, Feusner J, Hammond D: Prognostic factors for central nervous relapse in acute lymphoblastic leukemia. Proc Am Soc Clin Oncol 1989 (8):218

124 Omura GA, Moffitt S, Vogler WR: Combination chemotherapy of adult acute lymphoblastic leukemia with randomized nervous system prophylaxis. Blood 1980 (55):199-203

125 Wiernik PH, Dutcher JP, Gucalp R, Markus S, Esterhay R, Schiffer C, Weinberg V, Paietta E, Garl S, Benson L: MOAD therapy for adult acute lymphocytic leukemia. Proc Am Soc Clin Oncol 1990 (9):205

126 Kantarjian HM, Walters RS, Smith TL, Keating MJ, Barlogie B, McCredie KB, Freireich EJ: Identification of risk groups for development of central nervous system leukemia in adults with acute lymphocytic leukemia. Blood 1988 (72):1784-1789

127 Glass JP, Van Tassel P, Keating MJ, Cork A, Trujillo J, Holmes R: Central nervous system complications of a newly recognized subtype of leukemia: AMML with a pericentric inversion of chromosome 16. Neurology 1987 (37):639-644

128 Wolk RW, Masse SR, Conklin R, Freireich EJ: The incidence of central nervous system leukemia in adults with acute leukemia. Cancer 1974 (33):863-869

129 Stewart DJ, Keating MJ, McCredie KB, Smith TL, Youness E, Murphy SG, Bodey GP, Freireich EJ: Natural history of central nervous system acute leukemia in adults. Cancer 1981 (47):184-196

130 Cassileth PA, Sylvester LS, Bennett JM, Begg CB: High peripheral blast count in adult acute myelogenous leukemia is a primary risk factor for CNS leukemia. J Clin Oncol 1988 (6):495-498

131 Sullivan MP, Moon TE, Trueworth R, Vietti TJ, Humphrey GB, Komp D: Combination intrathecal therapy for meningeal leukemia. Two versus three drugs. Blood 1977 (50):471-479

132 Band PR, Holland JF, Bernard J, Weill M, Walker M, Rall D: Treatment of CNS leukemia with intrathecal cytosine arabinoside. Cancer 1973 (32):744-748

133 Wang JH, Pratt CB: Intrathecal arabinosyl cytosine in meningeal leukemia. Cancer 1970 (25):531-534

134 Simone JV: Treatment of meningeal leukemia. J Clin Oncol 1984 (2):357-358

135 Kun LE, Camitta BM, Mulhern RK, Laver SJ, Kline RW, Casper JT, Kamen BA, Kaplan BM, Barber SW: Treatment of meningeal relapse in chilhood acute lymphoblastic leukemia: 1. Results of craniospinal irradiation. J Clin Oncol 1984 (2):359-364

136 Land VJ, Thomas PRM, Boyett JM, Glicksman AS, Culbert S, Castleberry RP, Berry DH, Vats T, Humphrey GB: Comparison of maintenance treatment regimens for first central nervous system relapse in children with acute lymphocytic leukemia. A pediatric oncology study group. Cancer 1985 (56):81-87

137 Cherlow JM, Steinherz P, Gaynon P, Tubergen D, Trigg M, Bleyer WA, Sather H, Novak L, Hammond GD: Craniospinal radiation for CNS leukemia at presentation: how high does the spinal dose need to be? Proc Am Soc Clin Oncol 1991 (10):239

138 Steinherz P, Mandell L, Meyers P, Tan C, Fuks Z: Periodic CNS reinduction and delayed craniospinal radiation in the treatment of CNS relapse in acute lymphoblastic leukemia. Proc Am Soc Clin Oncol 1990 (9):221

139 Sariban E, Edwards B, Janus C, Magrath I: CNS involvement in American Burkitt's lymphoma. J Clin Oncol 1983 (1):677-681

140 Haddy TB, Adde M, Magrath IT: CNS involvement in small non cleaved-cell lymphoma is CNS disease per se a poor prognostic sign. J Clin Oncol 1991 (9):1973-1982

141 Liang R, Chiu E, Loke SL: Secondary central nervous system involvement by non-Hodgkin's lymphoma: the risk factors. Hematol Oncol 1990 (8):141-145

142 Nkrumah FK, Neequaye JE, Biggar R: Intrathecal chemoprophylaxis in the prevention of central nervous system relapse in Burkitt's lymphoma. Cancer 1985 (56):239-242

143 Anderson JR, Wilson JF, Jenkin RDT, Meadows AT, Kersey J, Chilcote RR, Coccia P, Exelby P, Kushner J, Siegel S, Hammond D: Childhood non-Hodgkin's lymphoma: the results of a randomized therapeutic trial comparing a 4-drug regimen (COMP) with a 10-drug regimen (LSA2-L2). N Engl J Med 1983 (308):559-565

144 Griffin J, Thompson RW, Mitchinson MJ, Kiewiet JC, Welland FH: Lymphomatous leptomeningitis. Am J Med 1971 (51):200-208

145 Bunn PA, Schein PS, Banks PM, De Vita VT: Central nervous system complications in patients with diffuse histiocytic and undifferentiated lymphoma: leukemia revisited. Blood 1976 (41):3-10

146 Ziegler JL, Blumming AS, Fass L, Morrow RJ: Intrathecal chemotherapy in Burkitt's lumphoma. Br J Med 1971 (3):508-512

147 Zuckerman KS, Skarin AT, Pitman SW, Rosenthal DS, Canellos GP: High-dose methotrexate with

citrovorum factor in the treatment of advanced non-Hodgkin's lymphoma. Blood 1976 (48):983-987
148 Rosen ST, Aisner J, Makuch RW, Matthews MJ, Ihde DC, Whitacre M, Glastein EJ, Wiernik PH, Lichter PH, Bunn PA: Carcinomatous leptomeningitis in small cell lung cancer. Medicine 1982 (61):45-53
149 Aroney RS, Dalley DN, Chan WK, Bell DR, Levi JA: Meningeal carcinomatosis is small cell carcinoma of the lung. Am J Med 1981 (71):26-32
150 Trump DL, Grossman SA, Thompson G, Murray K, Wharam M: Treatment of neoplastic meningitis with intraventricular thiotepa and methotrexate. Cancer Treat Rep 1982 (66):1549-1551
151 Giannone L, Greco F, Hainsworth JM: Combination intraventricular chemotherapy for meningeal neoplasia. J Clin Oncol 1986 (4):68-73
152 Stewart DJ, Maroun JA, Hugenholtz H, Benoit B, Girard A, Richard M, Russell N, Huebsch L, Drouin J: Combined intra-omaya methotrexate, cytosine arabinoside, hydrocortisone and thio-Tepa for meningeal involvement by malignancies. J Neurol Oncol 1987 (5): 315-322
153 Pfeffer MR, Wygoda M, Siegal T: Leptomeningeal metastases treatment results in 98 consecutive patients. Is J Med Sc 1988 (24): 611-618
154 Nakagawa H, Murasawa A, Kubo S, Nakajima S, Nakajima Y, Izumoto S, Hayakawa T: Diagnosis and treatment of patients with meningeal carcinomatosis. J Neurol Oncol 1992 (13):81-90
155 Sullivan MP, Viett TJ, Haggard ME, Donaldson MA, Krall JM, Gehan EA: Remission maintenance therapy for meningeal leukemia: intrathecal methotrexate versus intravenous bis-nitrosoureas. Blood 1971 (38):680-688
156 Willoughby MLN: Treatment of overt CNS leukaemia. In: Mastrangelo R, Poplack DG, Riccardo R (eds) Central Nervous System Leukemia: Prevention and Treatment. Martinus Nijhoff, Boston 1983 pp 113-122
157 Muriel FS, Schere D, Barengal: Remission maintenance therapy for meningeal leukemia: intrathecal and dexamethasone versus intrathecal craniospinal irradiation with radiocolloid. Br J Haematol 1976 (34):119-127
158 Humphray GB, Kron HF, Filler J: Treatment of overt CNS leukemia. Am J Pediatr Hematol Oncol 1972 (1):37-47
159 Frankel LS: The curative potential of CNS relapse in childhood acute lymphocytic leukemia. Proc Am Soc Clin Oncol 1982 (1):124

Evaluation and Management of Metastatic Spinal Cord Compression

Charles J. Vecht

Department of Neurology, Dr. Daniel den Hoed Cancer Centre, P.O. Box 5201, 3008 AE Rotterdam, The Netherlands

Metastatic spinal cord compression is a frequent complication which occurs in 5-10% of all patients with cancer [1]. As the immediate danger of spinal cord compression is irreversible paraplegia and incontinence, timely diagnosis and treatment are crucial. The most common cause of epidural cord compression is osseous metastasis to the vertebrae and any patient with vertebral metastasis runs a potential risk of development of damage to the spinal cord. Pain and a radiculopathy are other consequences of vertebral metastases and may develop alone or in combination. As these complications have many points in common for diagnostic workup and management, metastatic spinal cord compression will be discussed in this chapter together with back pain and radiculopathy in the cancer patient.

Presenting Signs

Pain

Any new pain in patients with cancer should be viewed with suspicion. Local pain secondary to vertebral metastasis as well as irradiating pain associated with a radiculopathy are common presentations of epidural metastasis leading to spinal cord compression. Pain is often considered as an almost obligatory sign of metastatic cord compression, but its incidence varies from 80% to 96% [1,3-9]. This implies that in patients who may have signs and symptoms of impending cord compression but without pain, a diagnosis of cord compression should not be ruled out. For example, epidural spinal cord compression due to osseous metastasis in prostate cancer is sometimes not associated with pain [10]. Compression of the thoracic cord is also fairly frequently seen without accompanying pain [1]. Nevertheless, pain is often the initial or only manifestation of beginning spinal cord compression. The pain can be local, it can be radicular or both. Local pain is often felt close to the site of the osseous metastasis, and is often perceived as continuous, dull or aching. An important feature of malignant pain from the vertebrae is that the pain gets worse at night or on lying down. A herniated disc is another common cause of back pain, but is usually more severe when the patient sits down.

On examination, about one-third of metastatic vertebrae are tender. At the same time, radicular pain may be present and is more common in cervical (79%) and lumbosacral regions (90%) than in the thoracic area (55%) [4]. Radicular pain can be uni- or bilateral; in the thoracic spine it is often bilateral. Occasionally the site of pain is misleading and can indicate referred pain. For example, when T12 or L1 vertebrae are affected, this may cause pain in the lower lumbar area [11]. Radicular pain often occurs in attacks and is felt as shooting pain. Also pain due to a lesion in the retroperitoneal space, for example para-aortic lymph-node metastasis in testicular cancer, can lead to pain in the lower spine which may or may not be associated with pain in the paravertebral dorsal region. Occasionally the pain is associated with Lhermitte's sign, which is characterised by a sensation of electric shock through the spine or both legs every time the patient bends his neck. This can occur in cervical as well as in thoracic cord compression. Also sneezing,

Table 1. Presenting signs of metastatic spinal cord compression

	%	Number
Pain	84	31/37
Paraesthesia	28	10/36
Sensory level	69	25/36
Ambulation grade *		
I	35	13/37
II	22	8/37
III	16	6/37
IV	14	5/37
V	14	5/37
Bladder dysfunction	47	16/34

* Ambulation was recorded as follows: grade I: walking independently; grade II: walking with aid is possible; grade III: walking impossible, both legs can be lifted from the bed, grade IV: muscle contractions in legs present, lifting of legs not possible; grade V: absence of contractions in legs [8]

coughing or movement can lead to an increase in pain and can be signs of osseous metastasis. Pain on movement may indicate instability of the vertebral column.

The duration of pain before other signs of spinal cord compression develop, may vary from 1 or 2 days up to many months, with a median interval from 6 weeks to 6 months [1,3,9,12]. Occasionally herpes zoster develops, usually unilateral and limited to 1 or 2 dermatomes which subsequently may be found to be the site of cord compression [1]. This association may be caused by activation of the latent virus by tumour involvement of posterior root ganglia.

Motor Weakness and Sensory Disturbances

Spinal cord compression often leads to paraparesis, which is seen in 64 to 85% of patients at the time of diagnosis [1,3-9] (Table 1).

The grade of weakness varies from still ambulatory at presentation in 11-57%, paraparetic but unable to walk in 30-74%, to paraplegia in 3-19% [3-5]. Tetraparesis in patients with spinal cord compression is rare and the majority of patients with a cervical metastasis present with radicular pain. Probably the relatively large diameter of the cervical canal compared to the thoracic spine provides more time for diagnosis and treatment once pain or radiculopathy start to develop, thus preventing frequent occurrence of cord compression at the cervical level.

An uncommon presentation of metastatic spinal cord compression is gait ataxia without any other associated symptom [3]. On examination an abnormal heel-to-knee-to-toe test is found without sensory symptoms and the patient may apparently suffer from cerebellar disease until cord compression is found. One assumes that the mechanism involves spinocerebellar tracts and we have observed this syndrome in patients with prostate cancer.

Sensory disturbances in patients with metastatic cord compression can be the consequence of radiculopathy or spinal cord damage. Symptoms of radiculopathy often start with a combination of paraesthesias, a subjective impression of diminished sensation or pain in the distribution of the affected roots. Signs of hypo-aesthesia, hypo-algesia or dysaesthesia are often found but rarely objective anaesthesia or analgesia, probably because usually only 1 or 2 roots are involved and overlap with areas innervated by more than 1 root is common. If cord compression develops, the patient often experiences a painless sensation of bilateral tingling or paraesthesia in both feet which either gradually or more rapidly rises up to legs and trunk. Also a feeling of tightness in both legs can be experienced. On examination one may find abnormalities of touch and position sense in the lower extremities indicating posterior tract dysfunction, together with disturbed sensation for pinprick and temperature sense if spinothalamic tracts are involved. As a rule, one finds an upper border of the sensory abnormalities on the trunk. This border indicates the level of the involved segments of the spinal cord. Because of the discrepancy between spinal cord segments and vertebrae due to the medullary ascensus, the involved vertebrae lie usually 2 or 3 vertebrae higher, causing compression of the spinal cord at the level of the corresponding dermatome. However, discrepancies between the suspected dermatome and affected vertebrae may occur due to changes in blood supply caused by arterial or venous occlusion or because observed radiologic abnormalities may be associated with asymptomatic involvement of the spinal cord.

Autonomic Disturbance

In an early stage, obstipation is a frequent sign of spinal cord damage. Later on it may lead to imperative micturition or urge incontinence. At the time of diagnosis of epidural cord compression, about half of the patients are incontinent due to bladder dysfunction [1,3,4,6-8].

Differential Diagnosis

On the whole, spinal cord compression usually shows a remarkably uniform clinical picture which is straightforward and usually not difficult to diagnose. Most patients have local pain in the spine with or without associated radicular pain together with painless pyramidal weakness of both lower legs, incontinence and a sensory level on the torso. If lumbar vertebrae are involved, the conus medullaris can be involved if metastases of the first and second lumbar vertebrae cause compression of this lowest part of the spinal cord. Mostly, lumbar vertebral metastases give rise to polyradiculopathy or cauda equina syndrome, with compression of one or more lumbar or sacral roots. In that case, there is usually local pain in the back together with irradiating pains in one or both legs in the distribution of affected roots. Motor weakness, if present, also indicates which roots are involved. Patients often suffer from incontinence which is characterised by obstipation and retention or a distended bladder. The marked discrepancy between spinal cord and cauda compression is that the first is characterised by severe, though painless, weakness in the legs and the second by often excruciating radicular pain in the legs with relatively intact motor function. Both have local pain in the spine in common.

The differential diagnosis of metastatic spinal cord compression in cancer patients includes extramedullary intradural metastasis, intramedullary metastasis, radiation myelopathy and radiation-induced secondary tumours. Other causes of spinal cord compression are cervical spondylotic myelopathy, epidural abscess in patients with bacterial discitis, tuberculosis of the spine, thoracic herniated disc, arteriovenous malformations and primary tumours of the spine or its contents, including neurinoma, meningeoma, ependymoma and astrocytoma.

The differential diagnosis of metastatic compression of the cauda equina also includes intradural drop-metastasis or meningeal carcinomatosis in cancer patients. Meningeal carcinomatosis of the lumbar or sacral roots often leads to reflex asymmetries, motor and sensory loss of involved roots, often without local pain in the spine or radicular pain. Of course, a herniated disc or narrowed lumbar canal are common causes of compression of one or more lumbar and sacral roots and this can also happen in patients with cancer.

Imaging studies

A diagnostic workup for suspicion of spinal cord compression should be performed as an emergency. Diagnosis includes demonstration of the lesion which causes the compression of the spinal cord but should also be aimed at providing information for defining the proper treatment, be it delineation of radiation fields or the need for biopsy or surgery. The diagnostic workup usually starts with plain X-rays of the symptomatic area or of the whole spine. In cancer patients with back pain and normal neurological examination, about 60% show vertebral metastasis on X-rays in the symptomatic area [2,13]. Patients with clinical signs indicating a radiculopathy or myelopathy have evidence of vertebral metastases on X-ray in 65% of cases [2,13]. Loss of more than half of bone material is necessary before lytic lesions show up in radiographs of lumbar vertebrae [14]. Therefore, plain X-rays can easily be false negative, and one will usually proceed with a Tc99m bone scan which is more sensitive for early detection of bony lesions [15]. However, bone scans have a significant false-positive rate for metastasis, particularly in patients with solitary abnormalities [16,17]. How should one proceed in patients with cancer - or a strong suspicion of it - who have normal radiographs and positive Tc99m bone scans? The use of spinal CT has demonstrated that one-third of such patients have benign disease and two-thirds have bony metastases [18]. If CT documents metastatic disease, one can detect with intrathecal contrast-enhanced CT that 25% of patients have epidural compression, although occupying less than half of the vertebral canal. In patients with a compressed vertebra on X-rays and positive bone scan, one-third have benign fractures and two-thirds have metastatic disease with 63% of the latter having epidural compression. If radiographs show metastasis without compression fractures, this is confirmed by spinal CT in almost all cases, with epidural compression present in about 50%, although none of these patients have any neurological abnormalities [18]. The presence of cortical bone discontinuity accentuates the risk of spinal cord compression, for in 65-91% this is associated with epidural compression as seen on spinal or intrathecal contrast CT [2,18,19].

In two-thirds of cases there is rostro-caudal extension of the epidural mass, without contiguity with cortical disrupted bone [19]. If epidural extension is found, local radiotherapy is worth considering [20].

Although CT can demonstrate the presence of epidural tumour, the advantage of myelography is that it more easily defines the rostral-caudal extent of the tumour and helps to delineate the proper radiation field. In one study with positive myelograms in cancer patients, half of the CT-scans were false negative although this study was performed at the time of second- or third-generation CT-scanners [21].

In patients exhibiting clinical signs of myelopathy, more than 75% have a myelographic block occluding more than 75% of the vertebral canal. A similar, extensive myelographic block is found in half of those with radiculopathy and in one-third of patients with only back pain and normal neurological findings [2,13]. In one study of male veterans with cancer who had only back pain together with a normal neurological examination, no epidural disease was found [13]. In cases of suspicion based on cord compression or radiculopathy, multiple epidural metastases are found in one-third of all cancer patients who undergo myelography [22]. This information is essential for delineating the proper radiation field, particularly if one realises that more than 16-25% of patients have tumour recurrence within the spinal canal just outside the original treatment field. More than half of these occur within a distance of 3 vertebrae from the initial epidural lesion and within a short time frame (4 months or less) following treatment of the initial lesion [23,24]. These data suggest that a large part of early recurrences within the spinal canal represent regrowth at the border of the radiation port. Designing larger radiation ports which encompass 2 vertebra instead of 1 above and below the level of compression might be a way to prevent most of these early epidural recurrences [24].

Patients with extracranial lymphoma present special problems. If they develop back pain without any other neurological sign and normal spine X-rays or bone scan, further workup including myelography may well demonstrate a complete block.

In general, if one performs a myelogram or intrathecal contrast-enhanced CT of the spine, a lumbar or cervical puncture is unavoidable. An advantage of this is that cerebrospinal fluid is obtained for laboratory examination including cytology. In patients with spinal cord compression as found on myelography, the protein content of the spinal fluid is often increased. An intrinsic risk of performing a lumbar puncture in patients with complete block in the spinal canal is the danger of spinal cord herniation. Removal of fluid under the block causes a pressure gradient over the block and may lead to a downward shift and increased pressure on the cord which can result in a partial or incomplete transverse lesion. This complication was already described by Elsberg [25] and later repeatedly confirmed by others [12,26,27]. One study has reported that 14% of patients with a complete myelographic block acutely deteriorated after lumbar puncture [28]. We believe that in clinical practice this deterioration may often go undetected as deterioration is the expected course for these patients, until treatment starts.

We think that in patients with a strong suspicion of metastatic spinal cord compression, lumbar puncture should possibly be avoided. Nevertheless, clinical judgement should determine whether it is needed to perform a spinal tap for suspected leptomeningeal disease or opportunistic infections of the central nervous system.

In order to demonstrate an epidural lesion, one can easily perform a descending myelogram via a C1-C2 lateral puncture which carries no risk for spinal herniation. As the majority of patients with metastatic spinal cord compression have a lesion in the thoracic spine, the procedure can be performed in the flat recumbent position with flexion of the head in order to avoid leakage of the contrast material into the intracranial cisterns. In this way there is no extra risk of intracranial contrast which can occur following contrast application via the lumbar route in case of an incomplete block and the patient is brought in Trendelenburg position in order to move the contrast to the thoracic and cervical regions.

If on descending myelography a complete block is found, the question arises if one should perform a lumbar puncture to delineate the lower level of the block. As this again implies the risk of spinal herniation, it is our choice to avoid it, if possible. Instead, one can perform an intrathecal contrast-enhanced CT by using the same contrast material injected for the cervical myelogram, in order to visualise the lower level of the block. If this gives insufficient information, we use an unorthodox method. Based on the combined information of plain radiographs of the upper level of the block and neurological picture, radiation ports are delineated and the patient receives dexamethasone followed by radiotherapy for 3 or 4 fractions. We feel that it is then justified to perform a myelogram by lumbar puncture to visualise the lower border of the block because one can assume that there is now less pressure on the spinal cord owing to previously applied treatment. On the basis of the outcome of the second myelogram, it is decided together with the radiotherapist if radiation ports need to be adjusted to encompass the lower border or other epidural deposits below the block.

Of course, these problems may soon be outdated, now that magnetic resonance is rapidly being introduced into clinical medicine. Particularly for accurate and non-invasive visualisation of the surroundings of the spinal canal and its contents, MR seems ideal. At present, myelography and MR are generally considered to be equal in their ability to detect epidural tumour blocking the spinal canal [29,30]. Smaller epidural lesions and root involvement still seem to be visualised better by myelography than by MR [30]. However, since the introduction of enhancement with Gadolineum-DTPA for spinal MR, this will probably become the standard evaluation for suspected epidural metastasis and subarachnoid spinal metastasis and may prove to be superior to myelography [31].

At this time, performing a myelogram for suspicion of metastatic spinal cord compression is still routine in many hospitals, because too little MR equipment is available for easy or instantaneous access to this technique. It also may happen that patients cannot undergo MR scanning because they are phobic, wear metal prostheses or have too much pain to lie down for longer periods. Therefore, it could be that for a minority of patients indications for myelography will continue to exist.

Treatment

Glucocorticosteroids

Glucocorticosteroids play an important role in the management of spinal cord compression. Experimental studies show that administration of corticosteroids leads to multiple effects. These include facilitation of neuronal excitability and nerve transmission, an increase in spinal blood flow by promoting vasodilatation by ß-receptor activation, impairment of vasoconstriction by inhibition of prostaglandin and thromboxane synthesis and lessening of peroxidation of neuronal cell membranes [32].

Experimental spinal cord compression leads to subsequent impairment of the vertebral venous plexus and vasogenic oedema. This is followed by autonomic dysregulation of spinal circulation, decrease in spinal blood flow and finally irreversible cord damage. Use of dexamethasone in a dose of 10 mg/kg in an experimental model of spinal cord compression gave significant but transient improvement in neurological function and a reduction of water content of the compressed spinal cord [33].

A reduction of the increased water content of compressed segments has also been observed with indomethacin, a non-steroidal anti-inflammatory drug, together with inhibi-

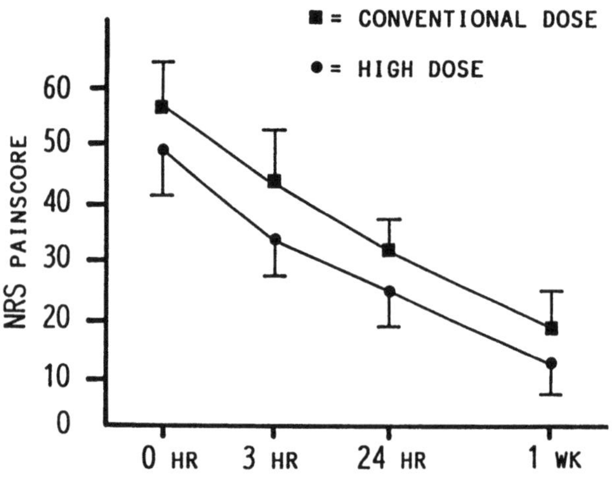

Fig. 1. Pain relief as determined by numerical rating scale (NRS) following initial treatment with 100 mg versus 10 mg i.v. bolus followed by 16 mg dexamethasone per day and radiotherapy [8]

tion of prostaglandin E_2 synthesis. Administration of both dexamethasone and indomethacin produced significantly fewer neurological signs than in control rats using an experimental model of neoplastic epidural spinal cord compression [34]. The vascular permeability as measured by Evans blue was significantly reduced by dexamethasone, methylprednisolone as well as indomethacin [36].

Comparisons between high- and low-dose dexamethasone in rats produced an equal but stronger improvement in neurological function when compared to untreated animals, although animal mortality was more frequent with high-dose dexamethasone because of infectious and gastrointestinal complications [37].

Based on these experiments, similar high-dose regimens have been applied in the clinical situation. One retrospective study using 100 mg i.v. bolus of dexamethasone followed by 96 mg per day for the first 3 days, followed by a tapering schedule, gave no indication of a better neurological improvement compared to conventional regimens, but it did seem to have a remarkable analgesic effect [4]. In the only randomised prospective trial available, an initial high dose of 100 mg i.v. following demonstration of complete block on myelography was found to be equally effective for the relief of pain as a conventional dose of 10 mg i.v. bolus, followed by 4 mg 4 times per day orally (Fig. 1). The effect of dexamethasone on pain for both the conventional and the high dose was substantial: 67% of patients improved remarkably within 24 hours. Also changes over time in neurological function were similar and there were no signs of any effect of these doses of dexamethasone in worsening or improving ambulation or bladder function [8].

The toxicity associated with high-dose regimens of dexamethasone can be considerable as observed in experimental and clinical studies, particularly when used for longer periods of time [6,37,38]. It is useful to realise that a conventional dose of dexamethasone of 16 mg daily is equivalent to 136 mg prednisone or 400 mg hydrocortisone daily. Given the absence of convincing positive effects for high-dose regimens and the observed toxicity, we favour a conventional schedule with an initial bolus of 10 mg dexamethasone i.v. followed by 16 mg per os daily.

Effect of Surgery and Radiotherapy

Treatment for metastatic spinal cord compression revolves around the issue of a combined neurosurgical and radiotherapeutical approach or radiotherapy alone. Surgery for metastatic spinal cord compression has been controversial since Elsberg [25] argued that there was no place for laminectomy for vertebral metastases. The other mainstay of treatment is radiotherapy and it is no surprise that many authors have compared the effect of both modalities. All studies conducted on this subject have been retrospective apart from one prospective trial, which, however, was so small in number and uneven in distribution, that no conclusion could be drawn [39]. Although a final estimation regarding the value of one approach over the other is not possible, we will review here the outcome of these studies.

Most reports have found that the pain is alleviated following treatment. The beneficial response to radiotherapy for pain varies from 69% to 94% [2,5,20,40,41]. Findlay has summarised these data in a review of 22 papers comparing a total of 1816 cases [42]. Based on these reports it was found that pain relief was achieved in 36% of patients following laminectomy, in 67% following combined laminectomy and radiotherapy and in 76% following radiotherapy alone with no significant differences between the latter 2 ways of treatment. A major outcome criterion is achieving ambulatory status following treatment but this favourable result depends to a large extent on the clinical status of the patient at the start of treatment. During the first week after treatment was started about 18% of patients improved, 58% remained stable and 24% deteriorated [8] (Fig. 2). On the whole, between 17 and 26% of patients deteriorated irrespective of which treatment was applied. Following laminectomy alone, 31% of patients who were paraparetic and 48% of patients who walked before treatment, became or remained ambulant. Following laminectomy and radiotherapy, 35% of paraparetic patients who were paraparetic before treatment and 67% of patients who walked before treatment, became or remained ambulant. Following radiotherapy alone, 42% of paraparetic patients and 79% of patients who walked before treatment became or remained ambulant [42].

If the patient keeps or regains his walking abilities following treatment, will he maintain ambulatory status? Of all walking patients post-treatment, 75% were still ambulant after 6 months [3]. In another study, of all walking patients, 87% of those who lived more than 1 year were ambulant and 73% of those living more than 2 years remained ambulant [6]. There is a sharp contrast in survival between walking and non-walking patients. In one prospective study the chance of surviving 1 year was 73% for ambulant patients and only 9% for patients not being ambulant after treatment [13].

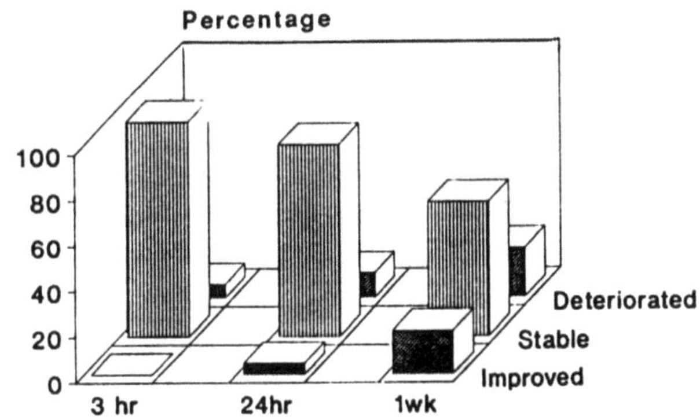

Fig. 2. The course of improvement in ambulation during the first weeks of treatment with dexamethasone and radiotherapy [8]

Uncertain Issues

One problem in management is whether there are differences between radiosensitive tumours (for example, lymphoreticular malignancies, breast, prostate and small cell cancer) and less radiosensitive tumours (including non-small cell lung cancer, renal cell cancer, melanoma and colorectal cancer). Patients with radiosensitive tumours who were paraparetic before treatment became ambulatory in 63% of cases following combined treatment with surgery and radiotherapy and in 40% if they suffered from less radiosensitive tumours. Following radiotherapy alone, 74% became ambulant with radiosensitive and 34% with less radiosensitive tumours [42]. As one multivariate analysis has demonstrated, the 2 determining factors for prognosis are motor function before treatment and the radiosensitivity of the tumour [9].

We believe that in paraparetic patients with radio-insensitive tumours, surgery is an option worth considering; this is a question ideally to be addressed in a prospective trial.

Another uncertain issue is what should happen with patients who are fully paraplegic before therapy can start. Findlay's review showed that patients become ambulant following laminectomy in 3%, following both laminectomy and radiotherapy in 7% and following radiotherapy alone in 2% [42]. In one study, 1 out of 8 paraplegic patients with radiosensitive tumours became ambulant following radiotherapy in contrast with 0 out of 20 patients with less radiosensitive tumours [3]. Another study reported on a group of 15 patients who had paralysis of both legs but still had varying levels of preserved sensation. Following radiotherapy, 5 patients from this group recovered ambulatory function either with or without the use of a cane, although the recovery was delayed for 3 months or more. Improved patients had either prostate, breast or small cell lung carcinoma [43].

How to treat rapidly progressing patients? Is it preferable that they undergo surgery first? A retrospective survey revealed that 55% (5 out of 9) of these patients deteriorated following surgery and radiotherapy, and 8% (1 out of 13) deteriorated following radiotherapy alone [3]. These figures would suggest that is not a mistake to treat rapidly progressing patients with radiotherapy alone, especially when radiosensitive tumours are involved.

Chemotherapy

Chemotherapy may occasionally be considered for metastatic spinal cord compression in patients with chemosensitive tumours, particularly non-Hodgkin's lymphoma, germ-cell tumours and possibly also breast carcinoma. Although there are no systematic studies on this subject, small series of patients or case descriptions have been reported [44-46].
We think that this approach may particularly be considered for patients with mild neurological abnormalities or asymptomatic epidural disease. One should realise that radiotherapy is also very effective for these tumours and that fractionation schemes for radiation of metastatic spine disease rarely lead to radiation myelopathy.

Anterior Decompression

A major obstacle for surgical decompression by means of laminectomy in metastatic spinal cord compression is the presence of the bulk of the tumour mass in the vertebral body. Anteriorly located metastases can hardly be reached via this route and only posterior decompression of the spine can be achieved. Another problem in using this approach is the immediate risk of an unstable spine, particularly if there is extensive destruction or compression fracture of the vertebral body. In these conditions the spine should be stabilised; this may involve technical difficulties with the posterior approach, although it is feasible [47]. As the majority of epidural metastases invade the vertebral column anteriorly, anterior decompression of the spine can be advantageous for removal of tumour tissue while leaving the vertebral arches intact. This method has been very successful in a selected group of patients with metastatic spinal cord compression [48]. Particularly patients with only 1 or 2 adjacent metastatic vertebrae and absent or stable tumour activity outside the spine are good candidates for this type of surgery. Usually the vertebral body is resected along with the epidural tumour and stabilisation is achieved with acrylate material and special rods which can be connected with healthy vertebrae above and below the excised body. Although it is hard to perform controlled studies evaluating the outcome of this procedure, the overall ambulation rate following treatment was 75% in one study with 85% of patients experiencing pain relief and a median survival of 8 months [49]. In another study, before treatment 11 patients were ambulatory and 24 paraparetic or paraplegic while at 1 month after surgery 28 patients were able to walk [50].

Conclusions

The outcome for patients with metastatic spinal cord compression is still based on early detection and treatment of the epidural tumour, as the functional status of the patient at the start of therapy determines to a large extent ambulatory status after treatment. Loss of ambulation is also associated with short survival. New developments in symptomatic treatment include the effect of non-steroidal inflammatory agents on spinal cord oedema and pharmacological prevention of neural tissue damage. It is still an unresolved issue under what conditions surgical treatment is needed, particularly for radio-insensitive tumours. A major step forward is the anterior surgical approach in selected patients with metastatic spinal cord compression. As treatment results improve, the issue of stability of the spine should also receive the attention it deserves.
A summary of guidelines for evaluation and treatment can be found on the next pages.

Acknowledgement

We thank Janet van Vliet for secretarial assistance.

Guidelines for the Evaluation and Management of Metastatic Spinal Cord Compression

In patients with suspicion of metastatic spinal cord compression,

start **dexamethasone** as 10 mg bolus intravenously,
followed by 4 x 4 mg intravenously or per os

followed by **emergency evaluation** according to guidelines below:

obtain X-ray,
 if negative, obtain bone-scan
 if positive, or if cancer is still suspected
obtain MRI scan,
or cervical (descending) myelography
 for assessment of cranio-caudal extension of epidural mass
 or for presence of multiple epidural deposits
followed by intrathecal contrast-enhanced CT of the spine
 for caudal extension if myelography shows complete block
 and for assessment of paravertebral expansion of tumour mass.

If this evaluation demonstrates that the lesion may well be a metastasis,
and the patient is **not known to have cancer:**

* obtain biopsy to verify tumour presence and further treatment approach,
* or perform laminectomy
* or anterior decompression with stabilisation of spine.

In patients known to have cancer:

Radiotherapy to the symptomatic spine is the main treatment
with radiation ports based on neuro-imaging studies.

Main Indications for Radiotherapy

for metastatic spinal cord compression include
* radio-sensitive tumours
* radio-insensitive tumours if patients are still ambulant
* rapidly progressing patients (?)
* following surgery (see below).

Laminectomy

(prior to radiotherapy) may be considered for:
* metastasis to posterior spine
* paraparetic patients with radio-insensitive tumours (?)
* in recurrent tumour following previous radiotherapy
* in progressing paraparesis despite ongoing radiotherapy
* patients not known to have cancer.

Anterior Surgical Approach

(excision of metastatic vertebral body with replacement
by acrylic material and stabilisation of the spine)
(prior to radiotherapy) may be considered if
* single or adjacent vertebral body metastasis is present and
* patients have an estimated survival of >1 year and
* no or stable extra-spinal tumour activity is present.

Alternative treatment with chemotherapy may be considered instead, or added to radiotherapy, in:
* non-Hodgkins's lymphoma
* multiple myeloma
* breast cancer
* germ cell tumours.

This particularly applies to asymptomatic epidural metastasis or if neurological signs are mild and not rapidly progressing so that radiotherapy can still be administered if the tumour is not responsive to chemotherapy.

Algorithm for **Back Pain only, in patients known to have cancer:**

obtain X-ray
obtain bone scan if X-ray is negative

(Note: one-third of single hot spots on bone scan in cancer patients are benign lesions)

If either one or both are convincing for vertebral metastasis:

radiotherapy may be applied

However, if information is still felt to be insufficient:

obtain MRI scan,

or cervical (descending) myelography followed by
intrathecal contrast-enhanced CT of the spine

in order to delineate tumour mass and radiation ports.

If X-ray and bone scan are negative, with still a strong clinical suspicion of metastatic disease:

obtain MRI

or cervical (descending) myelography, followed by
intrathecal contrast-enhanced CT of the spine

in order to detect and delineate tumour mass for radiation ports.

Radiculopathy in patients known to have cancer:

obtain X-ray
obtain bone scan if X-ray is negative

(Note: one-third of single hot spots one bone scan in cancer patienst are benign lesions)

obtain MRI

or cervical (descending) myelography
with intrathecal contrast-enhanced CT of the spine

in order to define mass
or detect multiple lesions for delineation of radiation ports.

REFERENCES

1 Barron KD, Hirano A, Araki S, Terry RD: Experiences with metastatic neoplasms involving the spinal cord. Neurology 1959 (9):91-106
2 Rodichok LD, Harper GR, Ruckdeschel JE: Early diagnosis of spinal epidural metastases. Am J Med 1981 (70):1181-1187
3 Gilbert RW, Kim JH, Posner JB: Epidural spinal cord compression from metastatic tumor: Diagnosis and treatment. Ann Neurol 1978 (3):40-51
4 Greenberg HS, Kim JH, Posner JB: Epidural spinal cord compression from metastatic tumor: Results with a new treatment protocol. Ann Neurol 1980 (8):361-366
5 Tang SG, Byfield JE, Sharp TR, Utley JF, Quinol L, Seagren SL: Prognostic factors in the management of metastatic epidural spinal cord compression. J Neuro Oncol 1983 (1):21-28
6 Martenson JA, Evans RG, Lie MR, Ilstrup DM, Dinapoli RP, Ebersold MJ, Earle JD: Treatment outcome and complications in patients treated for malignant epidural spinal cord compression. J Neuro Oncol 1985 (3):77-84
7 Nubourgh Y, Nguyen TH, Brihaye J, Lustman J, Gillard A, De Neve W: Les Métastases épidurales au niveau du rachis. Etude clinique de 82 cas. Acta Nuerol Belg 1985 (95):44-56
8 Vecht ChJ, Haaxma-Reiche H, Van Putten WLJ, De Visser M, Vries EP, Twijnstra A: Initial bolus of conventional versus high-dose dexamethasone in metastatic spinal cord compression. Neurology 1989 (39):1255-1257
9 Kim RY, Spencer SA, Meredith RF, Weppelmann B, Lee JY, Smith JW, Salter MM: Extradural spinal cord compression: analysis of factors determining functional prognosis. Prospective study. Radiology 1990 (176):279-282
10 Liskow A, Chang CH, Desanctis P, Benson M, Fetell M, Housepian E: Peidural cord compression in association with genitourinary neoplasms. Cancer 1986 (58):949-954
11 Foley KM: Pain syndromes in patients with cancer. In: Bonica JJ, Ventafridda V (eds). Advances in Pain Research and Therapy, Vol. 2. Raven Press, New York 1979 pp 59-75
12 Botterell EH, Fitzgerald GW: Spinal cord compression produced by extradural malignant tumours: early recognition, treatment and results. Canad M A J 1959 (80):791-806
13 Ruff RL, Lanska DJ: Epidural metastases in prospectively evaluated veterans with cancer and back pain. Cancer 1989 (63):2234-2241
14 Edelstyn GA, Gillespie PJ, Grebbell FS: The radiological demonstration of osseous metastasis: experimental observations. Clin Radiol 1967 (19):158-162
15 Citrin DC, Bessent RG, Greig WR: A comparison of the sensitivity and accuracy of the Tc-99 phosphate bone and skeletal radiograph in the diagnosis of bone metastases. Clin Radiol 1977 (28):107-117
16 Pistenma DA, McDougall R, Kriss JP: Screening for bone metastases, are only scans necessary? JAMA 1975 (231):45-50
17 Corcoran RJ, Thrail JH, Kyle RW et al: Solitary abnormalities in bones, scans of patients with extraosseous malignancies. Radiology 1970 (121):663-667
18 O'Rourke T, George CB, Remond J et al: Spinal computed tomography and computed tomographic metrizamide myelography in the early diagnosis of metastatic disease. J Clin Oncol 1986 (4):567-583
19 Weissman DE, Gilbert M, Wang H, Grossman SA: The use of computed tomography of the spine to identify patients at high risk for epidural metastases. J Clin Oncol 1985 (3):1541-1544
20 Redmond J, Friedl KE, Cornett P, Stone M, O'Rourke T, George CB: Clinical usefulness of an algorithm for the early diagnosis of spinal metastatic disease. J Clin Oncol 1988 (6):154-157
21 Anand AK, Krol G, Deck MDF: Lumbosacral epidural metastases: CT evaluation and compraison with myelography. Comp Radiol 1983 (6):351-354
22 Van der Sande JJ, Kröger R, Boogerd W: Multiple spinal epidural metastases: an unexpected frequent finding. J Neurol Neurosurg Psychiat 1990 (53):1001-1003
23 Loeffler JS, Glicksman AS, Tefft M, Gelch M: Treatment of spinal cord compression: A retrospective analysis. Med Pediatr Oncol 1983 (11):347-351
24 Kaminski HJ, Diwan VG, Ruff RL: Second occurrence of spinal epidural metastases. Neurology 1991 (41):744-746
25 Elsberg CA: Surgical Diseases of the Spinal Cord, Membranes and Nerve Roots. P.B. Hoeber, New York 1941 p 501
26 Mullan J, Evans JP: Neoplastic disease of the spinal extradural space. Arch Surg 1957 (74):900-909
27 Vecht ChJ, van Doorn JL: The risk for spinal herniation in spinal cord compression: lumbar or cervical myelography? Ned T Geneesk 1985 (129):171-174
28 Hollis PH, Malis LI, Zappulla RA: Neurological deterioration after lumbar puncture below complete spinal subarachnoid block. J Neurosurg 1986 (64):253-256
29 Smoker WAK, Godersky JC, Donzelli R et al: The role of MR imaging in evaluating metastatic spinal disease. AJNR 1987 (8):901-908
30 Hagenau C, Grosh W, Currie M, Wiley RG: Comparison of spinal magnetic resonance imaging and myelography in cancer patients. J Clin Oncol 1987 (10):1663-1669
31 Blews DE, Wang H, Ashok J, Robb PA, Phillips PC, Bryan RN: Intradural spinal metastases in pediatric patients with primary intracranial neoplasms: Gd-DTPA enhanced MR vs CT myelography. J Comp Assist Tomography 1990 (14):730-735
32 Hall ED, Braughler JM: Glucocorticoid mechanisms in acute spinal cord injury: a review and therapeutic rationale. Surg Neurol 1982 (18):320-327
33 Ushio Y, Posner R, Posner JB, Shapiro W: Experimental spinal cord compression by epidural neoplasms. Neurology 1977 (27):422-429
34 Siegal T, Shohami E, Shapiro Y, Siegal Tx: Indomethacin and dexamethasone treatment in experimental neoplastic spinal cord compression:

Part 2. Effect on edema and prostaglandin synthesis. Neurosurg 1988 (22):334-339
35 Siegal T, Siegal Tz, Shapira Y, Sandbank U, Catane R: Indomethacin and dexamethasone treatment in experimental neoplastic spinal cord compression: Part 1. Effect on water content and specific gravity. Neurosurg 1988 (22):328-333
36 Siegal T, Siegal Tz, Lossos F: Experimental neoplastic spinal cord compression: Effect of anti-inflammatory agents and glutamate receptor antagonists on vascular permeability. Neurosurg 1990 (26):967-970
37 Delattre JY, Arbit E, Rosenblum MK, Thaler HT, Lau N, Galicich JH, Posner JB: High dose versus low dose dexamethasone in experimental epidural spinal cord compression. Neurosurg 1988 (22):1005-1007
38 Weissman D, Dufer D, Voge V, et al: Corticosteroid toxicity in neuro-oncology patients. J Neuro Oncol 1987 (5):125-128
39 Young RF, Post EM, King GA: Treatment of spinal epidural metastases. Randomized prospective comparison of laminectomy and radiotherapy. J Neurosurg 1980 (53):741-748
40 Maranzano E, Latini P, Checcaglini F, Ricci S, et al: Radiation therapy in metastatic spinal cord compression. A prospective analysis of 105 consecutive patients. Cancer 1991 (67):1311-1317
41 Cobb CA, Leavens ME, Eckles N: Indications for nonoperative treatment of spinal cord compression due to breast cancer. J Neurosurg 1977 (47):653-658
42 Findlay GFG: Adverse effects of the management of malignant spinal cord compression. J Neurol Neurosurg Psychiat 1984 (47):761-768
43 Helweg-Larsen S, Rasmusson B, Soelberg Sorensen P: Recovery of gait after radiotherapy in paralytic patients with metastatic epidural spinal cord compression. Neurology 1990 (40):1234-1236
44 Oviatt DL, Kirshner HS, Stein RS: Successful chemotherapeutic treatment of epidural compression in non-hodgin's lymphoma. Cancer 1982 (49):2446-2448
45 Cooper K, Bajorin D, Shapiro W, Krol G, Sze G, Bosl GJ: Decompression of epidural metastases from germ cell tumors with chemotherapy. J Neuro Oncol 1990 (8):275-280
46 Boogerd W, Van der Sande JJ, Kröger R, Bruning PF, Somers R: Effective systemic therapy for spinal epidural metastases from breast carcinoma. Eur J Cancer Clin Oncol 1989 (25):149-153
47 Cybulski GR: Methods of surgical stabilization for metastatic disease of the spine. Neurosurgery 1989 (25):240-252
48 Siegal T, Siegal Tz, Robin G, et al: Anterior decompression of the spine for metastatic epidural cord compression: A promising avenue of therapy? Ann Neurol 1982 (11):28-34
49 Sundaresan N, Galicich JH, Lane JM, et al: Treatment of neoplastic epidural cord compression by vertebral body resection and stabilization. J Neurosurg 1985 (63):676-684
50 Siegal T, Siegal Tz, Robin G, Fuks Z, Yosipovitch Z. C1 Spinal cord compression by malignant epidural tumors: Results of anterior vertebral body resection. Ann Neurol 1983 (14):110

Lesions of the Peripheral Nervous System

Jerzy Hildebrand

Service de Neurologie, Hôpital Erasme, Route de Lennik 808, 1070 Brussels, Belgium

The identification of peripheral nervous lesions plays at least two important roles in the management of cancer patients: a) by allowing an earlier diagnosis of the underlying neoplasia and thus hastening its therapy, or b) by pointing to new locations of an already known malignancy and thereby determining its extent.

Treatment of peripheral nervous system lesions in cancer patients first requires the determination of their pathogenesis. These lesions are caused most commonly by metastases or local spread of malignancy. They may also be related to anticancer treatments including surgery, radiation therapy and chemotherapy. Less frequently are they the result of a remote effect of cancer. Finally, peripheral nervous lesions may be due to causes unrelated to cancer which are beyond the scope of this review.

This chapter will deal with cranial nerve lesions, plexopathies, mononeuritis multiplex and peripheral neuropathies. Spinal root lesions found in meningeal carcinomatosis and epidural metastases will be considered in the chapters by D. Gangji and Ch. Vecht.

Cranial Nerve Lesions

From a diagnostic point of view, it is convenient to distinguish 3 main locations of cranial nerve lesions: the base of the skull, the head and neck, and the root of the neck and the mediastinum.

Lesions at the Base of the Skull

These lesions are primarily due to metastases which originate from osteolytic cancers such as carcinomas of the breast, lung, prostate, kidney and thyroid or myelomas. In an analysis of 43 patients with cranial nerve dysfunctions due to metastases, Greenberg et al. [1] have identified 5 syndromes which are summarised in Table 1.

Table 1. Main symptoms and signs due to base of the skull metastases

Syndromes	Symptoms	Signs and nerves involved
Orbital)) Parasellar)	- unilateral frontal pain - diplopia	Exophthalmos (orbital) III - IV - VI (ptosis, diplopia) vein turgescence (parasellar)
Middle fossa	- facial numbness or pain	Vb, Vc (sensory); sometimes: VII - III - IV - VI
Jugular foramen	- post auricular pain - glossopharyngeal neuralgia - hoarseness, dysphagia	IX, X, XI (atrophy weakness: of palate, vocal cords, trapezius, sternocleidomastoid, tongue)
Occipital condyle	- occipital pain	XII; neck stiffness

Adapted from Greenberg et al. [1]

Whilst in many cases these syndromes overlap, particularly the last two, their distinction provides a usefull guidance for the radiological investigations searching for skull metastases. However, even if bone lesions are found in areas unrelated to the neurological features, they are indicative of the metastatic nature of the cranial nerve dysfunction.

The main differential diagnoses of cranial nerve lesions due to skull metastases are meningeal carcinomatosis, brain stem metastases, and lesions unrelated to cancer such as Bell's palsy, Miller-Fischer or Tolosa-Hunt syndromes. In the absence of peripheral polyneuropathy, cranial nerve lesions due to chemotherapy are very rare but have been reported [2,3]. Taking into account the differential diagnosis, an algorithm represented in Table 2 is proposed for patients with cranial nerve lesions.

Cancer patients developing cranial nerve lesions should have skull X-ray, isotopic scan and/or CT-scan. If these examinations demonstrate bone metastases, radiation therapy is initiated. If not, lumbar puncture and MRI scan with gadolinum should be performed to rule out leptomeningeal or parenchymal metastases or to prove skull metastases.

In patients without known cancer who develop cranial nerve palsies, a series of examinations aiming to find an underlying neoplasia should be performed. If this is found, local radiation therapy plus other appropriate anticancer therapies are then given. In patients with a negative workup, a careful follow-up is required. Metastases may mimic several "idiopathic" syndromes. For instance, the clinical presentation of metastatic tumours developing in cavernous sinus may resemble the Tolosa-Hunt syndrome, including its response to corticosteroids. One of the best examples illustrating the discrepancy between the benignancy of the clinical presentation and the severity of prognosis of isolated cranial nerve lesions is provided by the report of

Table 2. Diagnostic and therapeutic algorithm in patients with cranial nerve lesions

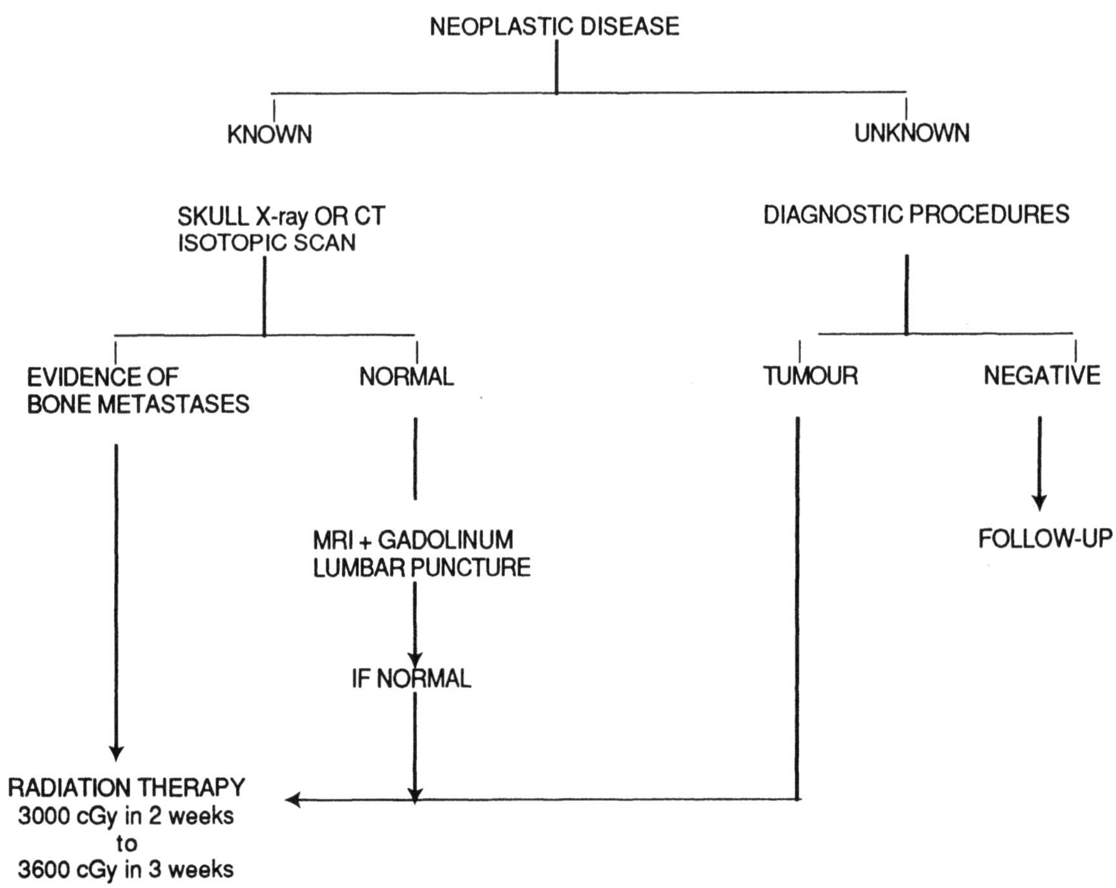

Massey et al. [4]. In 9 of their 19 patients mental neuropathy (numb chin syndrome) was the presenting symptom of a neoplasm, and despite the benignancy of the clinical presentation, 16 patients died within 17 months. The differential diagnosis may be particularly difficult in, admittedly, rare cases, where cranial nerve dysfunction is caused by peripheral spread of cutaneous squamous cell carcinoma [5]. In such cases normal radiologic findings or healing of the skin lesions may delay the diagnosis.

Therapy

Standard radiation therapy consists of 3000 cGy given in 10 fractions, but higher doses may be used to treat particularly aggressive tumours. This treatment alleviates symptoms in over 80% of cases, however, objective improvements of the neurological deficits are less common, especially in patients in whom the symptoms were present for more than 1 month prior to the initiation of radiotherapy [1].

Head and Neck Lesions

The clinical presentations of the epidermoid carcinoma of the nasopharynx have been analysed by Turgman et al. [6]. This interesting study reports a 9-year nationwide Israeli experience. In their initial stages, these tumours are notoriously silent, and 23 of 74 patients started with neurological signs. Eventually, half of the patients presented with neurological complications of which 92% were limited to cranial nerve dysfunction. The Rosenmüler fossa is a favourite site of origin of these tumors from which they tend to enter the cranial cavity through the foramen laceratum. Potentially every cranial nerve can be impaired, the most commonly involved being the VIth (68%) and the Vth (65%).
Other tumours causing cranial nerve lesions at the neck level are either thyroid, laryngeal, tongue or paranasal sinus carcinomas, sarcomas, lymphomas, or metastatic tumours. Neurological signs are often unilateral and involve the IXth through the XIIth cranial nerve. In these patients the most difficult differential diagnosis concerns lesions due to radiation therapy. In a single-institution series Berger and Bataini [7] observed 35 post-radiation cranial nerve lesions in 25 patients who had received 6000 cGy or more, 12 to 100 months prior to the development of the cranial nerve neuropathy. The nerves most commonly involved were the XIIth (19 times), followed by the Xth (9 times), XIth (5 times) and Vth (once).

Therapy

The management of cranial neuropathies caused by head and neck neoplasia depends on the nature of the tumour. It includes surgery, radiation therapy, chemo- and hormone therapy. In the vast majority of cases, radiation therapy will be used as the initial symptomatic treatment. As in the treatment of skull-base metastases, this treatment should not be delayed, because objective remission of cranial nerve palsies are inversely correlated with the delay prior to irradiation [8].

Lesions of the Root of the Neck and the Mediastinum

The main peripheral nervous structures involved at this level are the recurrent laryngeal nerve, the phrenic nerve and the cervical orthosympathic ganglion. Combinations of lesions of these structures lead to 3 main syndromes which are useful for an early diagnosis of mainly lung carcinomas.
The syndrome combining a lesion of the left recurrent laryngeal nerve, which loops around the arch of the aorta, with a paralysis of the left phrenic nerve points to a usually metastatic enlargement of the lymph nodes of the carina.
The combination of the right recurrent laryngeal nerve, which loops around the subclavian artery, with right phrenic nerve dysfunction, indicates a lesion at the apex of the right lung. Horner's syndrome is common in these patients.
Pancoast's syndrome is almost invariably indicative of a lung carcinoma located in the pulmonary superior sulcus. Its first manifestation is a reported pleural pain, often an aching sensation, located at the anterior aspect of the chest and the shoulder. Subsequently, sensory and motor symptoms and signs are due to the involvement of the eighth cervical and first and second thoracic root segments.

Horner's syndrome is frequently found [9,10] and often suggests epidural spread of the tumour.

Therapy

When patients with a Pancoast's syndrome are treated in early stages (pain in the shoulder), presurgical radiation therapy followed by excision of the neoplastic lesion yields approximately 30% survival at 5 years. Conversely, in patients with involvement of the brachial plexus and/or lymph nodes the prognosis for cure or long-term survival becomes dismal [11]. However, radiation therapy and surgery often relieve the pain [12]. Patients with persisting pain should undergo spinal MRI or myelography to rule out epidural neoplastic infiltration. In fact, in many centres these investigations are part of the standard workup of any Pancoast's syndrome.

Plexopathies

The treatment of a plexopathy developing in cancer patients naturally requires the determination of its aetiology. Although brachial and lumbosacral plexopathies will be considered separately, the main and most arduous differential diagnosis in cancer patients in both situations, is cancerous versus post-radiation injury. Other causes such as acute brachial neuritis or trauma are less common and generally easy to identify.

Brachial Plexophathy

Both cancerous and post-radiation brachial plexopathies are associated with the same malignancies, primarily lung and breast carcinomas and less frequently lymphomas. Table 3 summarises the clinical parameters which should be taken into account in making the differential diagnosis [13,14]. Cancerous lesions are about 10 times more common than post-radiation plexopathies. The latter require, of course, a history of radiation therapy, and their incidence is related to the dose and size of irradiation fields. However, even the accepted doses of 5000 cGy given in 25 fractions or 4500 cGy in 20 fractions carry a low but definite risk of about 3%. The delay between cancer diagnosis or irradiation and the onset of plexopathy ranges from months to over 20 years and is of no help in the differential diagnosis. A predominance of signs in the lower trunk in cancerous plexopathy and in the upper trunk in radiation plexopathies has been reported [13] but is not a constant finding. Though the progression rate is more insidious and sometimes self-limiting in radiation plexopathies, this feature is of no real help in early stages when the differential diagnosis is to be made. Finally, the presence of referred nerve pain as the initial symptom and sign of tumour recurrence are the most

Table 3. Differential diagnosis between cancerous and post-radiation brachial plexopathies

Parameter	Cancerous	Post-radiation
Incidence	10 times more common	Dose-related
Initial symptom	Pain in over 90%	Numbness, paraesthesia, pain in less than 20%
Signs	Predominantly lower trunk	Predominantly upper trunk
Progression rate	Slow	Insidious, self-limiting
Latency	Months to over 20 yrs mean: several years	
Tumour progression	CT: focal lesions in over 90%	CT: loss of planes, no focal lesions
EMG		Myokimia (motor unit bursts)

reliable indications of cancerous lesions. In the vicinity of the brachial plexus, neoplastic recurrence is best demonstrated by CT [14] or MRI scans (Fig. 1). These two procedures and/or myelography may also demonstrate epidural lesions as the neoplastic tissue tends to spread along the nerve roots. If doubt persists, biopsy should be performed; it is a safe procedure when carried out carefully [15]. However, a negative exploration does not rule out a neoplastic origin.

Lumbosacral Plexopathies

Unlike brachial plexopathies, the primary tumours associated with cancerous or post-radiation plexopathies differ. Colorectal carcinomas, sarcomas and lymphomas are most frequently associated with cancerous lumbosacral plexopathies [16,17]. Cervical and ovary primaries predominate in post-radiation plexopathies. The use of bilateral radiation fields in the treatment of these cancers accounts for the predominantly bilateral, yet often asymmetrical, distribution of post-radiation lumbosacral plexopathies. Thus, the nature of the primary tumour and the bilateral, versus unilateral, distribution are an indication as to the nature of lumbosacral plexopathy. But the most reliable features in favour of cancerous plexopathy (see Table 4) are again the presence of referred nerve pain as the initial symptom, and the evidence of local signs of tumour recurrence on CT or MRI scans (Fig. 2). Electrophysiological studies are of limited value but the occurrence of myokimia with motor unit bursts has been reported in both brachial and lumbosacral post-radiation plexopathies [18].

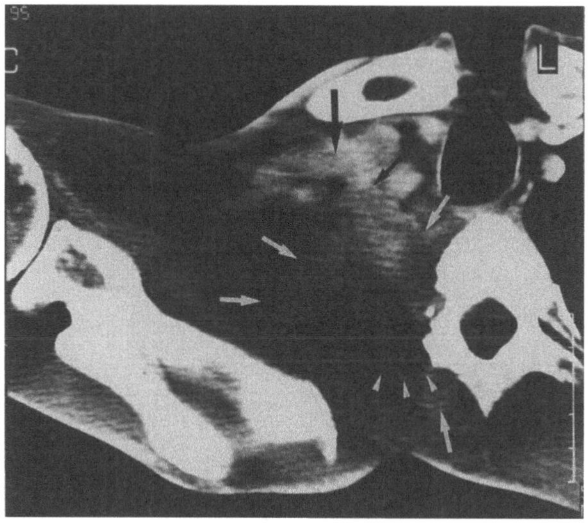

Fig. 1. CT-scan showing tumor involvement of the right brachial plexus by a small cell carcinoma of the lung. The neoplastic right apical mass (white arrows) causes an osteolytic lesion of the transverse process of a thoracic vertebra (white arrow heads) and extends to the brachial plexus (small black arrow) and the subclavian vein (large black arrow). (Courtesy M. Lemort, M.D.)

Table 4. Differential diagnosis between cancerous and post-radiation lumbosacral plexopathies

Parameter	Cancerous	Post-radiation
Primaries	**Colorectal**, sarcomas, lymphomas, breast carcinoma	**Cervical**, ovarian carcinoma Dose-related
Initial symptom	Pain in 70 to 80%	Weakness in about 50%
Signs	Bilateral in 10 to 25%	Bilateral in 80%
Latency	Variable	Median 5 yrs 1 to 31 yrs
Tumour progression	Focal CT (MRI) abnormalities	No focal abnormalities
EMG		Myokimia (motor unit bursts)

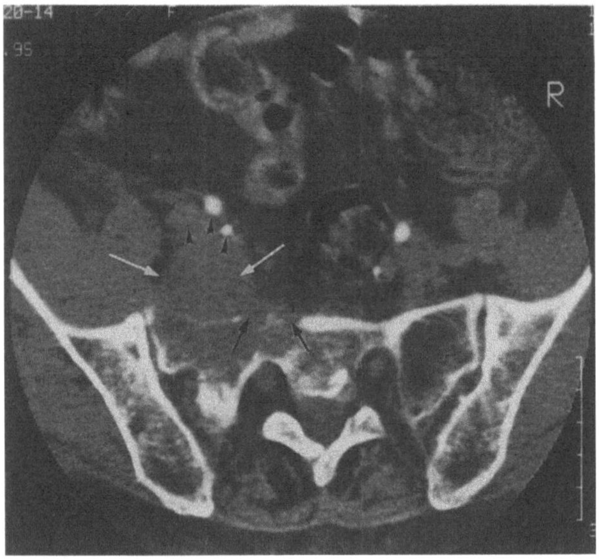

Fig. 2. CT-scan performed in a patient with a non-Hodgkin's lymphoma invading the left aspect of the sacrum and the presacral space (white arrows) and causing cortical bony disruption. Note the anterior displacement of the left iliac vessels and ureter (black arrow heads). (Courtesy M. Lemort, M.D.)

Therapy

The treatment of post-radiation plexopathies is disappointing. It has been suggested that decompressive surgery consisting in liberation of nervous structures from the surrounding fibrosis may be benificial. Practically, however, the procedure is seldom performed and is potentially hazardous since it may put at risk the already compromised blood supply of the nervous trunks. Cancerous plexopathy, especially pain, responds to radiation therapy if and when it can still be used. This treatment is often consolidated by chemo- and hormone therapy adapted to the nature of the primary malignancy.
Despite the administration of specific antineoplastic treatments, pain may persist as a major therapeutic challenge. In cancerous plexopathy pain may be generated in the periphery by chemical or mechanical stimuli, or be due to abnormal afferent impulses, including deafferentation pain. Non-narcotic analgesics act primarily on the former mechanism, whereas narcotics are effective on the latter. Adjuvant drugs such as tricyclic antidepressants may be useful.
If systemically administrated drugs fail, local approaches may be useful. These techniques, which require specialised skills, include:
a) neurosurgical interruption at the level of the dorsal roots (rhizotomy), dorsal ganglia entry zone (spearing motor fibres), or lateral columns (cordotomy). The latter technique is most useful in unilateral nociceptive pain below the waist;
b) chemical lesions of spinal roots using intrathecal or epidural injection of phenol or ethanol. These procedures are less selective and may cause significant weakness;
c) epidural or intrathecal injection of low doses of narcotics (morphine) by means of a continuous infusion system;
d) electrical stimulation of dorsal columns or thalamus. Both techniques are best indicated in deafferentation pain but are rarely very effective in cancer patients.

Peripheral Nerve Lesions

Peripheral polyneuropathy, mononeuritis and moneuritis multiplex are more common in cancer patients than in the general population. The 2 forms of peripheral nerve lesions differ, however, not only with regard to their clinical presentation but also in their aetiology, and therefore will be considered separately.

Peripheral polyneuropathies

Three clinically distinct presentations of peripheral neuropathies are seen in cancer patients with an increased frequency: a) the dying back polyneuropathy; b) the sensory neuronopathy and c) the Guillain-Barré-like polyradiculoneuritis.
The dying back neuropathy is the most common form of peripheral neuropathy in cancer patients as well as in the general population. Its causes are primarily toxic and metabolic. In cancer patients specifically, they may be due to the neurotoxicity of chemotherapeutic agents [19] or to the remote effect of cancer on the nervous system [20] (Table 5).
With the exception of the late stages of acute leukaemia [21], neoplastic infiltration of peripheral nerves is unlikely to produce symmetrical dying-back type polyneuritis.
The sensory neuronopathy may be caused by the administration of cisplatin [22] or taxol

Table 5. Cancer-related causes of peripheral neuropathies

Syndrome	Neoplastic compression or infiltration	Anticancer chemotherapy	Paraneoplasia
Dying back polyneuropathy	Very rare, seen in acute leukaemias	Vinca alkaloids Procarbazine Hexamethylamine	Most common form of neurological paraneoplasia
Sensory neuropathy	-	Cisplatin Taxol	Denny-Brown sensory neuronopathy
Guillain Barré-like syndrome	Meningeal carcinomatosis	Suramin	Associated with lymphomas, mainly Hodgkin's disease

[23], or be a paraneoplastic manifestation occurring either in isolation [24] or as part of a more widely-spread paraneoplastic syndrome including limbic encephalitis, cerebellar and brain stem dysfunction.

Meningeal carcinomatosis sometimes produces a Guillain-Barré-like syndrome. The latter also seems to occur with an increased frequency in lymphomas, mainly Hodgkin's disease, where it is considered to be a paraneoplastic manifestation [25].

Therapy

Withdrawal of the neurotoxic chemotherapy is justified only when the neuropathy becomes disabling. However, it must be remembered that symptoms and signs of peripheral neuropathy associated with cisplatin or vincristine treatments may progress after drug discontinuation. Prevention of chemotherapy-induced neuropathy includes avoiding the co-administration of other, even mildly neurotoxic, drugs [26] and possibly the co-administration of several potentially useful substances.

Thus, glutamic acid has been shown to decrease the severity of vincristine-induced neuropathy in mice and also in a randomised and double-blind clinical trial [27]. The most significant effect was on the prevention of loss of Achilles tendon reflexes and paraesthesias. The mechanism by which glutamic acid inhibits vincristine neurotoxicity is unknown, but it does not seem to affect its antineoplastic activity.

A mixture of gangliosides (Cronassial) exerts a favourable preventive effect in experimental models by partially preventing both electrophysiologic [28] and morphologic changes in peripheral nerves, but its effectiveness in humans has not been established (Fig. 3).

In mice, nerve growth factor prevents the neurotoxic effects of vinblastine in sympathetic ganglia [29], of taxol in dorsal root ganglion neurons *in vitro* [30], and of the experimental cisplatin neuronopathy [31].

The prevention of cisplatin neurotoxicity by an ACTH analogue (ORG 2766) first found in animals has been tested in the clinic by Gerritsen van der Hoop et al. A dose-related protective effect was demonstrated in women treated with cisplatin and cyclophosphamide for ovarian cancer. The threshold of vibration perception was the main parameter used to measure the neurotoxicity [32].

Mononeuritis and mononeuritis multiplex

The diagnostic and therapeutic problems raised by mononeuritis and mononeuritis multiplex are similar to those previously considered for cranial nerve lesions. They may be either the presenting sign of a malignancy or, when diagnosed in cancer patients, indicate a new spread of the disease. Their clinical presentation is that of an asymmetrical, randomly distributed sensory-motor peripheral deficit, and the main causes in cancer patients other than neoplastic involvement are: a) paraneoplastic vasculitis; b) post-radiation fibro-necrosis; c) haematomas, which are often found in acute leukaemias or in patients with blood coagulation disorders; d) toxicity of paravenous injections or local perfusions with neurotoxic drugs [33].

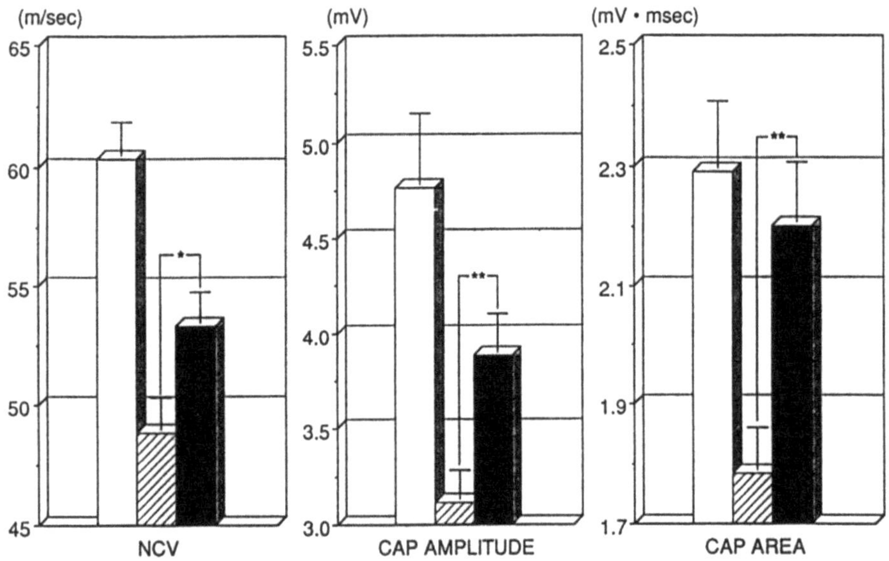

Fig. 3. Nerve conduction velocity (NCV) and compound action potential (CAP) recorded in rabbit sciatic nerve after a 5-week treatment with 0.20 mg/kg vincristine per week without gangliosides (dashed bars) or with 50 mg/kg per day of Cronassial given i.v. (solid bars). Age-matched control animals (empty bars) received saline phosphate buffer. (Courtesy M.G. Fiori, M.D.)

Lambert-Eaton Syndrome

Two-thirds of Lambert-Eaton Syndrome (LES) cases are associated with cancer, primarily small cell lung carcinoma (SCLC). LES is a rare disease. Even in the selected group of SCLC patients, its incidence is lower than 2%. In the majority of cases the diagnosis of LES precedes the discovery of the underlying neoplasia.

LES is characterised by proximal weakness which starts and predominates in the lower limbs, causing difficulties in climbing stairs or even standing up from a sitting position. Unlike in myastenia gravis, the oculo-bulbar musculature is usually speared. Signs of cholinergic dysautonomia are present in about 50% of cases.

The diagnosis is confirmed by electrophysiological features which include: a) a low compound muscle action potential (CMAP); b) a decrease in CMAP amplitude at low-frequency (<5 Hz) repetitive stimulation, and c) an at least 2-fold increase in CMAP amplitude at high-frequency (20 to 50 Hz) stimulation. This typical pattern, however, is not observed in all cases [34].

LES is an autoimmune disease caused by antibodies directed against voltage-sensitive calcium channels. These channels are also expressed on the surface of the SCLC (but not on other lung cancers), thus generating an autoimmune reaction which down-regulates the calcium channels of the presynaptic nerve terminals.

Therapy

Therapy of LES combines different approaches aiming to a) decrease the tumour volume; b) increase the liberation of acetylcholine (ACH) packets, or c) inhibit the autoimmune reaction.

a) Reduction of tumour volume may improve the clinical and electrophysiological signs of the syndrome. LES is indeed the only paraneoplastic neuropathy which has been shown to improve, admittedly in a limited number of cases, after the cure of the underlying cancer [35-38].

b) At least 2 drugs which increase the liberation of ACH packets have been successfully used in LES therapy. Guanidine chlorohydrate 30 mg/kg in 3 to 4 daily fractions [39], and 3-4 diaminopyridine 15 to 25 mg total dose given in 4 to 5 daily doses [40]. Acetylcholinestherase inhibitors are ineffective in LES, but prostigmine potentiates the activity of 3-4 diaminopyridine [41]. The main side effects of these drugs are haematological, liver, and/or renal toxicity for guanidine and seizures for 3-4 diaminopyridine.

c) The effect of immunodepressive treatment using corticosteroids [42] and drugs such as azathioprine [43] may be delayed [42], thus limiting their use in cancer patients with short life expectancy. In addition, possible adverse effects of chronic administration of corticosteroids and cytotoxic drugs further limit their usefulness.

Plasmapheresis is also effective in LES but it is followed by an only short-term clinical response [43].

Summary

The vast majority of peripheral nervous lesions seen in cancer patients are caused by neoplastic spread.

Surgery is useful, and sometimes even curative, in rare cases such as early stages of Pancoast's syndrome.

Radiation therapy remains the mainstay in the treatment of these complications. It relieves pain more often than neurological deficits, and should not be delayed by unnecessary investigations since its effectiveness is inversely correlated with the duration of neurological symptoms.

Peripheral nerve lesions being signs of progression of the underlying neoplastic disease, focal radiation therapy is often supplemented by systemic treatments such as chemo-, hormone and/or immune therapy.

The most arduous differential diagnosis of cancerous peripheral neuropathies concerns post-radiation injuries, which do not respond properly to surgical decompression. Pain, which is often a predominant feature in these patients, may not respond to specifically antineoplastic treatments and must be managed vigorously, sometimes by means of specialised techniques.

REREFERENCES

1 Greenberg HS, Deck MDF, Vikram B et al: Metastasis to the base of the skull: Clinical findings in 43 patients. Neurology 1981 (31):530-537

2 Sandler SG, Tobin W, Henderson ES: Vincristine-induced neuropathy. Neurology 1969 (19):367-374

3 Whitaker JA, Griffith IP: Recurrent laryngeal nerve paralysis in patients receiving vincristine and vinblastine. Br Med J 1977 (1):1251-1252

4 Massey EW, Moore J and Schold SC: Mental neuropathy from systemic cancer. Neurology 1981 (31):1277-1281

5 Clouston PD, Sharpe DM, Corbett AJ et al : Perineural spread of cutaneous head and neck cancer. Arch Neurol 1990 (47):73-77

6 Turgman J, Braham J, Modan B and Goldhammer Y: Neurological complications in patients with malignant tumors of the nasopharynx. Europ Neurol 1978 (17):149-154

7 Berger PS and Bataini JP: Radiation-induced cranial nerve palsy. Cancer 1977 (40):152-155

8 Meyer JE and Wang CC: Carcinoma of nasopharynx. Factors influencing results of therapy. Radiology 1971 (100):385-388

9 Layzer RB: Neoplastic Diseases. In: Neuromuscular Manifestations of Systemic Disease. Davis Co, Philadelphia 1985, pp 258-259

10 Hepper NGG, Herskovic T, Witten DM et al: Thoracic inlet tumors. Ann Intern Med 1966 (64):979-989

11 Attar S, Miller JE, Satterfield J et al: Pancoat's tumor: Irradiation or surgery? Ann Thorac Surg 1979 (28):578-586

12 Batzdorf U and Brechner VL: Management of pain associated with the Pancoast' syndrome. Ann J Surg 1979 (137):638-646

13 Kori SH, Foley KM, and Posner JB: Brachial plexus lesions in patients with cancer: 100 cases. Neurology 1981 (31):45-50

14 Cascino TL, Kori S, Krol G, and Foley KM: CT of the brachial plexus in patients with cancer. Neurology 1983 (33):1553-1557

15 Bagley FH, Walsh JW, Cady B et al: Carcinomatous versus radiation-induced brachial plexus neuropathy in breast cancer. Cancer 1978 (41):2154-2157

16 Thomas JE, Cascino TL, and Earle JD: Differential diagnosis between radiation and tumor plexopathy of the pelvis. Neurology 1985 (35):1-7

17 Jaeckle KA, Young DF and Foley KM: The natural history of lumbosacral plexopathy in cancer. Neurology 1985 (35):8-15

18 Aho I, Sainio K: Late irradiation-induced lesions of the lumbosacral plexus. Neurology 1983 (33):953-955

19 Hildebrand J: Peripheral neuropathy. In: Hildebrand J (ed) Neurological Adverse Reactions to Anticancer Drugs. European School of Oncology Mongraph Series. Springer-Verlag, Berlin 1991 pp 93-99

20 Hildebrand J and Coërs C: The neuromuscular function in patients with malignant tumors. Brain 1967 (90):67-82

21 Krendel DA, Albright RE and Graham DG: Infiltrative polyneuropathy due to acute monoblastic leukemia in hematologic remission. Neurology 1987 (37):474-477

22 Roelofs RI, Hrushesky W, Rogin J, Rosenberg L: Peripheral sensory neuropathy and cisplatin chemotherapy. Neurology 1984 (34):934-938

23 Lipton RB, Aptel SC, Dutcher JP et al: Taxol produces a predominantly sensory neuropathy. Neurology 1989 (39):368-373

24 Denny-Brown D: Primary sensory neuropathy with muscular changes associated with carcinoma. J Neurol Neurosurg Psychiat 1948 (11):73-87

25 Lisak RP, Mitchell M, Zweiman B et al: Guillain-Baré syndrome and Hodgkin's disease. Three cases with immunologic studies. Ann Neurol 1977 (1):72-78

26 Hildebrand J, Kenis Y: Additive toxicity of vincristine and other drugs for the peripheral nervous system. Acta Neurol Belg 1971 (71):486-491

27 Jackson DV, Wells HB, Atkins JN et al: Amelioration of vincristine neurotoxicity by glutamic acid. Ann J Med 1988 (84):1016-1022.

28 Favaro G, Di Gregorio F, Panozzo C and Fiori MG: Ganglioside treatment of vincristine-induced neuropathy. An electrophysiologic study. Toxicology 1988, 49:325-329

29 Menesini MG, Chen JS, Calissano P and Levi-Montalcini R: Nerve growth factor prevents vinblastine destructive effects on sympathetic ganglia in newborn mice. Proc Natl Acad Sci 1977 (74):5559-5563

30 Apfel SC, Lipton RB, Arezzo JC and Kessler JA: Nerve growth factor prevents toxic neuropathy in mice. Ann Neurol 1991 (29):87-90

31 Apfel SC, Arezzo JC, Lipson LA and Kessler JA: Nerve growth factor prevents experimental cisplatin neuropathy. Ann Neurol 1992 (31):76-80

32 Gerritsen van der Hoop R, Vecht CJ, Van der Burg MEL et al: Prevention of cisplatin neurotoxicity with an ACTH (4-9) analogue in patients with ovarian cancer. N Engl J Med 1990 (322):89-94

33 Castellanos AM, Glass JP, Yung WKA: Regional nerve injury after intra-arterial chemotherapy. Neurology 1987 (37):834-837

34 Oh SJ: Diverse electrophysiological spectrum of the Lambert-Eaton myasthenic syndrome. Muscle & Nerve 1989 (12):464-469

35 Ongeboer de Visser BW, Boven E, and Ten Bokkel-Huinink WB: Lambert-Eaton syndrome: Electrophysiological normalization during chemotherapy. Clin Neurol Neurosurg 1979 (81):235-240

36 Jenkyn LR, Brooks PL, Forcier et al: Remission of Lambert-Eaton syndrome and small cell anaplastic carcinoma of the lung induced by chemotherapy and radiotherapy. Cancer 1980 (46):1123-1127

37 Clamon GH, Evans WK, Sheperd FA et al : Myasthenic syndrome and small cell carcinoma of the lung. Variable response to antineoplastic therapy. Arch Intern Med 1984 (144):999-1000

38 O'Neil JH, Murray NMF and Newsom-Davis J: The Lambert-Eaton myasthenic syndrome: a review of 50 cases. Brain 1988 (111): 577-596

39 Oh SJ and Kim KW: Guanidine hydrochloride in the Lambert-Eaton syndrome. Electrophysiological improvement. Neurology 1973 (23):1084-1090

40 McEvoy KM, Windeback AJ, Daube JR and Low PA: 3, 4-Diaminopyridine in the treatment of Lambert-Eaton myasthenic syndrome. N Engl J Med 1989 (321):1567-1571

41 Lundh H, Nilson O and Rosen I: Treatment of Lambert-Eaton syndrome: 3,4-diaminopyridine and pyridostigmine. Neurology 1984 (34):1324-1330

42 Streib EW and Rothner AD: Eaton-Lambert myasthenic syndrome: Long-term treatment of three patients with prednisolone. Ann Neurol 1981 (0):448-453

43 Newson-Davis J and Murray NMF: Plasma exchange and immunodepressive drug treatment in the Lambert-Easton myasthenic syndrome. Neurology 1984 (34):480-485

Supportive Care of the Neuro-Oncology Patient

Jerome B. Posner

Department of Neurology, Memorial Sloan-Kettering Cancer Center, 1275 York Avenue, New York, NY 10021, USA

Patients with cancers, particularly those affecting the nervous system, frequently suffer from disabling symptoms, some of which are only indirectly related to the cancer (Table 1). Some examples include pain, asthenia, fatigability, loss of appetite, and depression. These symptoms, which are often more distressing to the patient than the tumour itself, often do not respond to treatment directed at the underlying neoplasm and, thus, must be treated independent of treatment of the neoplasm.

As therapy for tumours involving the nervous system becomes more effective, the problems of dealing with symptoms that may result from therapy or irreversible destruction of vital structures by the tumour loom ever larger. A new field of supportive care and symptom management has developed for the treatment of cancer patients. The field publishes a journal (The Journal of Pain and Symptom Management) and has specialists at cancer hospitals who deal solely with supportive care and symptom management. Many of the symptoms requiring supportive care are found in patients suffering from neuro-oncological problems.

In patients with neuro-oncological illnesses, the symptoms requiring supportive care generally have 4 major causes: 1) The tumour itself may cause direct symptoms by destroying or compressing nervous system structures. Examples include headache from brain tumours, back and neck pain of vertebral metastases (with or without epidural spinal cord compression) and the pain caused by invasion of peripheral structures such as the brachial plexus. 2) The tumour may also cause indirect symptoms (i.e., paraneoplastic). Examples are the asthenia, fatigability and general malaise often associated with small neoplasms and thought to be caused by cytokines, such as cachexin, elaborated by the tumour or cells of the immune system responding to the tumour. 3) Symptoms requiring supportive care may be a side effect of treatment directed at the tumour. Both radiation therapy and chemotherapy with cytotoxic agents may have substantial side effects, particularly when these agents are directed at the nervous system. In addition, however, and virtually unique to neuro-oncology, there are the problems associated with side effects of drugs used for symptom relief rather than treatment of the underlying tumour. The major examples are corticosteroids for the treatment

Table 1. Symptoms in 240 patients with cancer

Symptom	No. pts. responding	Percentage pos. response
Fatigue	236	74.2
Worry	230	70.9
Sadness	236	66.1
Pain	236	62.7
Drowsiness	236	61.0
Dry mouth	237	56.5
Insomnia	240	53.7
Poor appetite	233	45.5
Nausea	238	44.5
Bloated	236	39.4
Difficulty concentrating	237	38.3
Constipation	227	33.5
Change in taste	230	36.5
Cough	237	30.4
Problems with sex	230	23.9
Incontinence	235	12.3
Nightmares	238	11.3

Portenoy, R. Unpublished data from Memorial Sloan-Kettering Cancer Center (with permission)

of brain and spinal cord oedema and anticonvulsants for the treatment or prevention of seizures. 4) Finally, psychological symptoms in response to tumours affecting the nervous system are often substantially greater than psychological symptoms in response to tumours affecting other parts of the body. There are two reasons for this. The first is that symptoms directly caused by tumours in the nervous system (e.g., aphasia, paralysis, incontinence) are substantially more devastating than, for example, the cough, pain and even shortness of breath produced by a lung tumour. Secondly, when the tumour involves the brain, particularly the frontal lobes, the damage it causes often decreases the ability of the patient to cope with the stress of having the disease; thus, a patient who might otherwise have the psychological reserve to deal with even a devastating illness loses some of that reserve when a portion of the brain is damaged.

This chapter discusses some of the problems associated with supportive care and symptom management in patients with neuro-oncological problems. The chapter emphasises the usefulness and side effects of drugs used not for the treatment of the primary tumour but for symptoms which arise as a direct or indirect effect of that tumour. Particular emphasis is placed on glucocorticoids and anticonvulsants.

Glucocorticoids

Glucocorticoid hormones are the most widely used drug in neuro-oncology. Their major use is for the control of brain and spinal cord oedema. However, steroids have several other important salutary effects which make them extremely useful in the supportive care of the cancer patient.

Salutary Effects

Steroids have been shown in controlled trials to increase the quality of life in pre-terminal or terminal cancer patients [1-4]. The drugs improve appetite and enhance the feeling of well-being in many patients. Steroids also appear to have substantial pain-relieving qualities [3]. The exact mechanism by which pain is relieved is not clear although the inhibition by steroids of release of nociceptive cytokines may play a role. In patients with spinal cord compression, pain relief is often dramatic and appears clinically to be independent of the relief of spinal cord oedema. Many patients with severe pain, when put on steroids, can decrease their intake of narcotics and, in some patients, relief of pain by steroids is more dramatic than that given by narcotics.

Steroids are also useful in the management of nausea and vomiting caused either by the cancer or its chemotherapy. A number of trials have documented the usefulness of corticosteroids either alone or in conjunction with other antiemetic agents in the control of chemotherapy-induced nausea and vomiting. In at least one of these studies the steroids also improved mood and sense of fatigue [5]. The mechanism by which steroids reduce nausea and vomiting is unknown but may be a direct effect of steroids on the vomiting centre of the brain-stem.

Corticosteroids are known to increase appetite as well as redistribute fat. In many instances, increase in appetite and weight gain are undesirable side effects of the steroids. However, this effect may be salutary in patients with terminal cancer [1]. Nevertheless, the increase in appetite and weight gain, even when they occur, are usually outweighed by the catabolic effects of steroids which increase fat but decrease muscle mass (see below). Other drugs, which may be effective in increasing appetite without the side effects of steroids, include cyprohepatidine [7], a serotonin antagonist, and high-dose megoestrol.

As many as half of the patients with cancer suffer at some stage of the disease from either asthenia, defined as a sensation of generalised weakness, easy tiring and decreased capacity for work despite no objective weakness in the individual muscles, or anorexia with or without cachexia, or both [8-10]. The pathogenesis of these abnormalities is unknown but increasing evidence suggests they result from increased cytokine production induced by the tumour. The implicated cytokines have included Interleukins-1 and 6 and Tumour Necrosis Factor-α [11].

The specific corticosteroid to use, its dose and the timing of doses are not established. Prednisolone, methylprednisolone and dexamethasone have all been used in various studies and yielded approximately comparable results. Relatively low doses of the drug (e.g., 32 mg of methylprednisolone daily) [1] appear to suffice but our experience suggests that in spinal cord compression, higher doses are necessary to control pain. Dexamethasone is widely used by neurologists in part for historical reasons but in part because its lack of mineralocorticoid effect obviates the salt retention sometimes induced by other corticosteroids. There are also differences in protein binding between prednisone and dexamethasone in that, at standard doses, less of the dexamethasone is bound. As a result, relatively more dexamethasone can be found in brain and CSF after systemic administration than prednisone. That difference has been suggested as the reason that acute leukaemia patients receiving dexamethasone have only one-half the number of meningeal relapses as those receiving prednisone [12].

The lack of mineralocorticoid effect is so complete that the physician must remember that in patients with adrenal failure associated with cancer (e.g., rare adrenal metastases or adrenalectomy), one cannot substitute dexamethasone for hydrocortisone without running the risk of volume depletion and vascular collapse [13].

There is at least one report suggesting that dexamethasone is less inhibiting to the migration of white cells into injured tissue and thus might be less immunosuppressive than other steroids [14]. On the other hand, the fluorinated steroids are believed by some to be more likely to produce steroid myopathy than non-fluorinated glucocorticoids [15].

Because patients with neuro-oncological problems treated with steroids are often receiving many other drugs, it is important for the physician to be aware of the interactions of steroids with other drugs. The most important interactions are with drugs that induce hepatic microsomal enzymes (cytochrome p450 system). Drugs such as phenytoin, phenobarbital and perhaps carbamazepine, increase the metabolic clearance of steroids and may decrease their therapeutic effect. One study suggests that the bioavailability of an oral dose of dexamethasone may be decreased to 20% of its previous bioavailability by the addition of phenytoin [16]. One result is that patients with brain tumours on stable doses of steroids may develop increased symptoms when they are coincidentally started on anticonvulsants. Phenobarbital has the same effect as phenytoin in increasing corticosteroid metabolism [18]. Conversely, one report [17] suggests that concomitant administration of dexamethasone may increase phenytoin levels. Our own experience has been the opposite. Many patients on stable doses of phenytoin may become toxic as the corticosteroid dose is decreased.

There is increasing evidence that corticosteroids are useful along with antibiotics in the treatment of meningitis and, indeed, some other infections such as pneumocystic pneumonia in the immunosuppressed host. Whether these same considerations apply in the cancer patient who suffers CNS infection is unclear. Corticosteroids may also suppress aseptic meningitis (probably caused by blood in the subarachnoid space) which sometimes follows neurosurgical procedures in primary or metastatic brain or spinal tumours.

Unwanted Effects of Steroids

Table 2 summarises some of the unwanted side effects of steroids. A number of reviews and most textbooks of pharmacology deal with these (and other) side effects of steroids [19-21]. Some of the more important ones for neuro-oncology are described in the paragraphs below.

Myopathy

Most patients who are given conventional doses (16 mg dexamethasone or equivalent) of steroids for more than 2 or 3 weeks develop at least mild steroid myopathy [22,23]. Histologically, there is bland atrophy of type-2 fibers. The syndrome is usually characterised by weakness of proximal muscles of the hip girdle with wasting of thigh muscles [24] so that patients have difficulty getting up from the toilet seat or from low chairs without pushing-off with their hands. If the disorder is more severe it may affect the ability to climb stairs or to lift heavy objects above the head [22,25]. At its most florid there is severe weakness of

Table 2. Side effects of steroids

Common but usually mild	Non-neurological but serious side effects
Insomnia	GI bleeding
Sensation of abdominal bloating	Bowel perforation
Increased appetite	Avascular necrosis (usually hip)
Visual blurring	Glaucoma
Urinary frequency and nocturia	Opportunistic infection
Acne	Hyperglycaemia
Oedema	
Exophthalmos	
Genital burning (IV push)	
Neurological side effects (common)	**Neurological side effects (uncommon)**
Myopathy	Psychosis
Behavioural alterations	Paraparesis
Hallucinations (high dose)	Seizures
Steroid withdrawal (see Table 3)	
Hiccups	
Tremor	
Visual blurring	

muscles of the neck (particularly the flexors), shoulder and pelvic girdle. The onset may be sudden and a few patients complain of myalgia. Less commonly there may be distal weakness and myalgia. Sensation is normal as are deep tendon reflexes. In some instances, respiratory function is compromised [22].

The differential diagnosis of proximal muscle weakness in patients on steroids includes metabolic and nutritional myopathies associated with cancer, leptomeningeal tumour producing predominantly proximal weakness, the Lambert-Eaton myasthenic syndrome, and polymyositis, the last two as remote effects of cancer. It is particularly important to consider polymyositis because this disorder is treated with steroids: the typical EMG changes of increased insertional activity, elevated muscle enzyme concentrations in serum and the histological findings of muscle necrosis or inflammation indicate myositis. These findings are almost always absent in patients with steroid myopathy. The treatment of steroid myopathy is discontinuation of the steroids, if possible, after which the myopathy usually resolves over time [27]. Anabolic steroids and B-complex vitamins, which have been reported to hasten resolution of steroid myopathy in experimental animals [28], do not appear to be effective in humans [27].

Steroid psychosis [29]

Psychotic changes associated with steroids were common when ACTH and naturally occurring glucocorticoids were more widely used. With synthetic steroids the disorders are less common and with dexamethasone florid steroid psychosis is rare. The Boston Collaborative Group reports the incidence of acute psychotic reaction to be 3% of patients treated with prednisone and to be dose-related [30]. However, a double-blind prospective trial of prednisone 80 mg daily for 5 days given to normal volunteers revealed that 11 of 12 patients developed at least mild psychiatric reactions during treatment or withdrawal [31]. Symptoms included irritability, anxiety, insomnia, trouble concentrating, euphoria or depression.

More severe psychiatric reactions are of 3 general types: affective, schizophrenic-like, and delirious [32]. A reversible dementia unassociated with symptoms of psychosis has also been reported [33]. Clonazepam has been used in the treatment of steroid-induced mania [34]. One group has suggested that divided doses of enteric coated steroid preparations increase the incidence of steroid-induced psychosis.

Affective disorders, either manic or, less likely, depressive psychosis (depression is more common with Cushing's syndrome than with exogenous steroid therapy), cannot be distinguished from the non-steroid associated psychiatric illness. The disorder usually begins early in the course of therapy, is more likely to affect females, and may be dose related. It resolves when the steroids are withdrawn. The disorder can be treated with neuroleptic drugs, but tricyclic drugs are not effective and may worsen symptoms. The disorder occasionally begins during tapering of steroids but resolves once the steroids are entirely discontinued. A persistent bipolar disorder after withdrawal of steroids has been described in one patient [35]. Three patients on alternate-day steroids have been reported to cycle with mood elevation on the on-days and depression on the off-days [36]. The phenomenon appeared to be dose related. A single report suggests that Lithium used prophylactically may prevent this form of steroid psychosis [37]. A history of steroid psychosis does not predict recurrent psychosis with a second course of steroids.

The second form resembles acute schizophrenia. The patient becomes withdrawn and/or paranoid and may experience auditory and/or visual hallucinations. The disorder cannot be distinguished from psychiatric illness and will respond either to withdrawal of steroids or to treatment with major tranquilizers.

The third form is acute delirium; the patient becomes distractible and unable to attend appropriately to environmental stimuli, confused and sometimes suffers visual hallucinations. Mild delirium is often not reported by the patient to the physician because the patient is neither surprised nor concerned about the hallucinations since he attributes them to the drug. The affective and schizophrenic-like steroid psychoses must be differentiated from a psychiatric disorder occurring in a patient under the stress of treatment for cancer. Delirium must be distinguished from other metabolic disorders which may complicate the cancer or its treatment.

Osteoporosis and avascular osteonecrosis

Osteoporosis, a common side effect of prolonged steroid use [38,39], is sometimes responsible for vertebral fractures. The back pain caused by vertebral fracture may lead the physician to suspect a vertebral tumour. Steroid-induced osteoporosis will reverse, at least in young persons, when the drug is discontinued [41]. Avascular osteonecrosis of the hips [40] (occasionally shoulders, wrist, clavicle) may be confused with spinal cord compression or peripheral neuropathy. Patients have usually been on steroids for a long time although there are occasional reports of patients developing osteonecrosis after only a few weeks of treatment [40]. There appears to be a correlation between dose and risk [42]. The hip disorder is characterised by pain in the hip, often radiating down the anterior aspect of the thigh to the knee and resembling, in some respects, a femoral neuropathy or lumbar radiculopathy. The pain causes difficulty in walking. The diagnosis can be made by reproducing the pain on rotation of the hip. In some patients, a click can be heard as the hip is passively flexed and extended. Early during the course of the disorder, plain X-rays, nuclide bone scans and CT scan may not be abnormal, but eventually they will reveal the necrosis. MRI is the most sensitive diagnostic test. One study suggests that a second-generation biphosphonate (APD) and calcium can prevent steroid-induced osteoporosis [43].

Lipomatosis

Steroids cause redistribution of fat. In most instances, fat redistributes to the face, causing the characteristic moon facies, to the abdomen producing a "pot belly" and, in many patients, a sensation of chronic abdominal bloating, and to the posterior lower neck causing the characteristic "buffalo hump". However, fat also redistributes to the retro-orbital space, sometimes causing proptosis, to the mediastinum and to the epidural space. Fat in the epidural space can cause the neurological signs and symptoms of spinal cord compression including paraplegia [44,45]. In some instances, surgical decompression of the cord has been necessary to relieve neurological symptoms. The typical fat density of the lesions in the epidural and mediastinal spaces on MR and CT scan can easily differentiate it from neoplasm.

Visual changes

Many patients receiving corticosteroids complain of visual blurring. The pathogenesis of this disorder is unknown but it appears due to change in refraction associated with the corticosteroids. The symptoms generally disappear as the steroids are tapered and discontinued. The visual system can also be affected by steroids in a number of other ways. Cataracts are common in patients on long-term steroids and have even been reported to be caused by intermittent dexamethasone use as an antiemetic [46]. Steroids can occasionally induce exophthalmos by increasing fat retro-orbitally [47]. They have been reported to induce mydriasis and ptosis in experimental animals [48] and may increase intraocular pressure leading to glaucoma [49].

Gastrointestinal dysfunction

Gastrointestinal (GI) bleeding and bowel perforation are two well-recognised complications of steroid therapy [50,51]. Although GI bleeding is generally considered more common, GI perforation is the more serious complication in neurological patients receiving steroids.

A major question is whether prophylaxis against GI ulceration and bleeding is useful in patients being treated with corticosteroids. There are little data to guide the physician. One study suggested that cimetidine was able to prevent the development of gastric ulcers induced by steroids in experimental animals [52]. A small double-blind placebo-controlled study in humans suggested that gastrointestinal symptoms and antacid consumption were lower in a group treated with cimetidine and steroids compared with those treated with placebo and steroids [53]. A study of patients with spinal cord trauma treated with either high-dose (Solu-Medrol 1 g a day) or low-dose (Solu-Medrol 160 mg a day) steroids and protected by either antacids alone or antacids and cimetidine, showed no difference in GI bleeding between the two groups. Unfortunately, there was no group which did not receive gastrointestinal prophylaxis. Incidentally, low-dose heparin did not affect the incidence of GI bleeding either, although full-dose heparin did [54].

The issue would be trivial were it not for the fact that gastrointestinal prophylaxis carries its own side effects. The H2 blockers have been associated with encephalopathy and have interactions with chemotherapeutic agents [53]. Alkalinisation with antacids leads to a significant increase in colonisation of Gram-negative bacteria in the stomach and the possible increase in aspiration pneumonia [55] and sucralfate binds a number of drugs in the stomach, preventing adequate absorption. As a result, it is my policy not to use gastrointestinal prophylaxis of any sort in patients on steroids unless there is a previous history of peptic ulceration. In that case, I prefer sucralfate, taking care that it is given at times different from other oral agents. At least one other neuro-oncologist agrees [56].

Bowel perforation generally affects the sigmoid colon [57,58]. The affected patients are usually constipated, often because of bowel dysfunction due to spinal cord compression. Clinical symptoms usually begin with moderate to severe pain in the abdomen but the physician is often misled because bowel sounds persist and rebound tenderness characteristic of peritonitis is often not present. The diagnosis can be made by finding free air under the diaphragm on upright abdominal or lateral decubitus films. The patient must be treated surgically although in a few instances bowel perforations apparently heal spontaneously. The risk is particularly high in patients treated for spinal cord compression because they are more prone to constipation. Prevention or early treatment of constipation (see below) might avert this serious complication. A more benign syndrome related to steroid therapy is pneumoptosis intestinalis. The air appears as cysts or linear streaks within the intestinal wall. The cysts may rupture but they heal spontaneously.

Miscellaneous side effects

Several other side effects of steroids (Table 2) are occasionally encountered in neuro-oncological practice. A particularly unpleasant one is hiccup [59,60] which appears to be a dose-related effect of corticosteroids in some patients. Treatment of steroid hiccup is often difficult unless the dose is decreased. However, phenothiazines, amphetamine, valproate and carbamazepine are sometimes

Table 3. Steroid withdrawal syndrome

Headache	Myalgia and arthralgia
Lethargy	Postural hypotension
Nausea, vomiting, anorexia	Papilloedema
Fever	

effective. Hypersensitivity and even anaphylaxis to corticosteroids have been reported [61,62] and occasionally patients develop psychological dependence on steroids [63]. A peculiar side effect of intravenous bolus injection of dexamethasone is a severe anogenital itching or tingling which is extremely distressing but generally subsides within a few minutes. The patient warned in advance of the possibility finds it tolerable [64,65].
Intrathecal administration of corticosteroids can cause a severe pachymeningitis [66,67]. Corticosteroids diminish both sense of taste and smell and can, on a few occasions, be a cause of relative anorexia [68].

Steroid withdrawal syndrome

Withdrawal of patients from steroids also causes neurological disability (Table 3) [69]. The most common symptom of withdrawal is so-called "steroid pseudorheumatism" [70,71]: patients develop acute myalgias and/or arthralgias which may be severe. One of our patients was admitted to the hospital with a presumptive diagnosis of spinal cord compression because severe pain in his legs impaired his ability to walk. In other patients, the disorder is milder and can be ameliorated by increasing the dose of steroids and tapering more slowly. Steroid pseudorheumatism usually follows rapid taper of steroids but, in a few of our patients, has occurred when the drug was decreased by as little as 2 mg a week. In those patients, each reduction seems to produce an exacerbation of the arthralgia which disappears over 36 to 48 hours.
Also common is a syndrome characterised by headache, lethargy and sometimes low-grade fever. The syndrome was first described by Amatruda [69] in patients who had no underlying neurological disease. It also occurs in patients with CNS disease and may lead the physician to believe the symptoms are due to recurrent brain tumour rather than steroid withdrawal. Withdrawal from prolonged steroid treatment in children has been reported to cause the syndrome of pseudotumour cerebri [72]. This finding may be a result of decreased CSF absorption when steroids are withdrawn [73]. Prolonged suppression of the hypothalamic pituitary adrenal axis may result in a true secondary adrenal insufficiency when steroids are tapered too rapidly; the disease often becomes clinically manifest when there is an intercurrent medical or surgical illness.
Because of their known immune suppressing capacities, steroids, whether exogenous or endogenous, can lead to opportunistic infections [74,75]. In the neuro-oncological setting, a common problem is opportunistic infection with pneumocystis carinii in patients who have been on steroids and are being tapered to lower doses [74]. Some have recommended prophylaxis with sulfamethoxazole/trimethoprim given as one double-strength tablet twice a day for 3 days each week. The drug is generally given to patients who are going to be on prolonged steroids and is discontinued a month after patients are off steroids.

Anticonvulsants

Seizures are frequent in patients with neuro-oncological disorders. About 20% of patients with brain metastases either present with or develop focal or generalised convulsions. The incidence is lower in patients with leptomeningeal metastases, vascular or infectious complications and the side effects of some cancer therapies. Seizures are common in primary brain tumours as well. Anticonvulsant agents all have potentially deleterious side effects and many have interactions with chemotherapeutic or other agents (e.g., glucocorticoids) used in the treatment of cancer. Thus, the decision to use anticonvulsants is not always an easy one. The physician must first consider whether to use anticonvulsant agents and, if the decision is positive, which agent to choose.
Most physicians treat patients with anticonvulsants if the patient has had a seizure. However, no studies address the question of

whether anticonvulsant agents prevent further seizures in patients with neurological complications of cancer even when blood levels of the agents are kept within accepted therapeutic range. Some evidence suggests no correlation between "therapeutic" serum phenytoin levels and partial seizures despite a correlation between such concentrations and generalised seizures [76]. Nonetheless, in the absence of proof, the use of anticonvulsant agents to prevent further seizures seems warranted.

The use of prophylactic anticonvulsants for patients at risk of having seizures is more controversial. One study failed to show a decrease in the incidence of seizures when patients with known metastases were treated with prophylactic anticonvulsants [77]. Another study suggests that prophylactic anticonvulsants prevent seizures in patients with cerebral gliomas [78]. The problem in many instances appears to be that it is difficult to maintain a therapeutic blood level especially in patients with metastatic cancer, at least in part because of interactions of anticonvulsants with anticancer agents. For example, several studies have shown that during the course of chemotherapy with BCNU, carboplatin and other drugs, the serum concentration of anticonvulsants decreases, presumably a result of microsomal enzyme induction [79-81] or decreased absorption [79]. Conversely, anticonvulsants such as phenytoin and phenobarbital may change the serum concentration of antineoplastic agents [82]. In occasional patients, a decrease in anticonvulsant serum concentration appears to be of clinical significance leading to seizures. To compound the problem, elevated levels of several of the anticonvulsant drugs cause toxicity which may mimic the symptoms of brain tumour or even cause increased seizure activity [83]. Thus, my policy is not to use prophylactic anticonvulsants in patients with brain metastases except in patients with malignant metastatic melanoma in whom, because of the predilection to involve gray matter, the incidence of seizures may be as high as 50%. I do use prophylactic anticonvulsants for patients with glioma [78].

If the physician decides to use anticonvulsant drugs, he must decide which of the drugs to use. In patients not on anticonvulsant drugs, who have or are suspected to have metastatic brain tumours and are about to undergo a contrast-enhanced CT scan, an oral prophylactic dose of a benzodiazepine (5 to 10 mg of diazepam 30 minutes before the procedure) decreases the incidence of seizures substantially [84]. Benzodiazepines are, likewise, the drugs of choice to abort a seizure. Given intravenously, the agents usually stop seizures promptly allowing time for slower acting standard anticonvulsants (e.g., phenytoin) to be given orally or intravenously.

For prophylaxis or long-term treatment of focal or generalised convulsions associated with systemic cancer, there are 4 major agents; phenytoin, carbamazepine, phenobarbital and valproate. Other less commonly used agents include primidone and clonazepam. There is little evidence that one drug is superior to another in the prevention of further seizures [85,86]. There is evidence that monotherapy, i.e., using maximally tolerated doses of a single agent, is superior to polytherapy (multiple agents) in the management of patients with epilepsy.

All anticonvulsant agents have side effects. Lethargy and cognitive dysfunction can be caused by any of the agents even when blood levels are within the "therapeutic" range. Recent evidence suggests that all anticonvulsant agents produce about the same degree of drowsiness and cognitive dysfunction [87,88]. However, carbamazepine and primidone, if given at full doses initially, produce profound drowsiness and may not be tolerated. These drugs must be started at low doses and gradually increased to reach appropriate levels. Both phenytoin and, less frequently, carbamazepine, have been reported to cause the Stevens-Johnson syndrome, particularly in the setting of patients receiving whole-brain radiation and on a decreasing dose of steroids [89]. If the patient has been on the anticonvulsant drug for more than a month without toxicity, steroid tapering and brain radiation appear to be safe. Phenytoin has been reported to produce granulomatous vasculitis and has, on occasion, caused pulmonary failure [90]; it has also been associated with osteomalacia [91]. In many patients on phenytoin, the level of alkaline phosphatase and other liver enzymes in the serum may be raised [92]. Involuntary movements, particularly choreoathetosis, may be a sign of phenytoin intoxication substituting for the more common ataxia and nystagmus [93].

Many patients taking carbamazepine complain of intermittent diplopia as well as drowsiness even at "therapeutic" doses. Carbamazepine lowers the white blood-cell count which may cause concern in patients being treated with myelosuppressive chemotherapeutic agents. However, true agranulocytosis from carbamazepine is rare and it is not clear that it potentiates the myelosuppression from chemotherapeutic agents.

In about 20% of patients with brain tumours in whom phenobarbital is used as a therapeutic agent, pain and dysfunction in the shoulder and sometimes the entire upper extremity (shoulder-hand syndrome) occur [94]. The shoulder-hand syndrome is usually contralateral to the site of the tumour and may occur even in patients who have no motor deficit.

Valproate has been reported to cause hepatic dysfunction in small children receiving multiple anticonvulsant agents [95]. It has also been reported to occasionally cause thrombocytopenia and to interfere with synthesis of coagulation factors such as fibrinogen. Since so many patients with neurological complications of cancer are on multiple drugs, I have been reluctant to use valproate although some clinicians have reported the drug to be safe and relatively efficacious. Occasionally, patients taking valproate will develop stupor or coma which clears when the valproate is discontinued. The syndrome may be a result of valproate-induced elevations of the blood ammonia level but the pathogenesis is not entirely known.

If anticonvulsants are used, the physician should probably follow blood levels on a periodic basis and certainly measure them any time an untoward effect might be related to the anticonvulsants. However, one should recognise that so-called "therapeutic levels" represent only guidelines. Many patients appear to have their seizures controlled at levels below the usual therapeutic range and many patients do not have signs of toxicity even at blood levels substantially above the therapeutic range. Thus, physicians are required to treat patients and not blood levels. Because of the long half-life of some of the drugs such as phenytoin, attempts to adjust phenytoin levels within the therapeutic range often lead to toxicity without altering the patient's propensity toward seizures.

For all of the reasons listed above, it is difficult to choose an anticonvulsant agent. All in all, the drug of choice is probably carbamazepine followed in order by phenytoin, valproate and phenobarbital. The failure of one of these agents does not predict the failure of the others. If seizures persist, switching to another drug may be efficacious. Phenytoin has the advantage of having both an intravenous and an oral preparation and of being amenable to loading for high-dose oral or intravenous treatment. There is no parenteral carbamazepine and, because of acute but transient drowsiness as a side effect, the drug must be started at low dose and increased slowly.

Anticoagulants

Most patients with cancer have concomitant disorders of coagulation [96]. In as many as 90% of cancer patients one may find circulating fibrinogen degradation products. Thrombophlebitis, with or without pulmonary embolus, is a major problem in patients with both primary and metastatic brain tumours, particularly those who undergo surgical treatment [97-99]. In addition to the general risk factor for thrombophlebitis in cancer patients, patients with brain lesions often suffer immobility of the extremities, predisposing to stagnation of venous blood and clotting. Even in patients without motor deficit, when thrombophlebitis develops it is twice as likely to occur in the extremity contralateral to a brain tumour, primary or metastatic, than in the ipsilateral limb [98].

Some precautions may decrease the incidence of thrombophlebitis, particularly in the postoperative period, in patients suffering from cancer. External pneumatic calf compression boots used both in the operating room and in the recovery room until the patient is fully ambulatory appear to substantially decrease the incidence of thrombophlebitis and pulmonary embolism [100]. The role of low-dose heparin in postoperative treatment is not clear [101] and many surgeons are reluctant to use it because of the possibility of intracranial bleeding. Low molecular weight heparin may prove to be safer and as efficacious [102].

When thrombophlebitis develops in the postoperative patient, or in a patient not operated on who has a known brain tumour, many physicians are reluctant to use therapeutic anticoagulation because of the fear of brain haemorrhage [103]. The fear appears to be poorly founded. In both patients with primary and metastatic brain tumours, there appears to be no greater incidence of haemorrhage into the tumour in patients anticoagulated than in those not treated with anticoagulants [98,104]. Thus, for patients more than 4 or 5 days postoperatively, or patients harbouring brain tumours who have not been operated on, thrombophlebitis should be treated as vigorously as it would be in a patient without a brain tumour. However, the use of anticoagulants in patients with or without cancer is not without risk. Heparin can induce thrombocytopenia and thrombosis [105] and warfarin can induce skin and sometimes breast, penile and toe necrosis [106]. Because of the risk of bleeding and these other complications of anticoagulants, many physicians place inferior vena cava filters to prevent pulmonary emboli in patients with cancer and lower extremity thrombophlebitis [107]. Although these filters appear to be effective, in our hands they seem occasionally to lead to massive oedema of the lower extremities which interferes with the patient's function. I prefer, when possible, to use anticoagulation with heparin followed by warfarin, reserving the Greenfield filters only for those patients in whom anticoagulation appears clearly contraindicated.

Analgesic Agents

Pain occurs in the majority of patients with end-stage cancer and is a particular problem in patients with epidural spinal cord compression and peripheral nerve invasion or compression. A vast literature addresses the problem of pain relief in patients with cancer [108] and only a few principles can be mentioned here. The major problem in providing adequate analgesia to patients with neurological complications of cancer is that the best analgesic drugs (i.e., narcotics) often add to the already present neurological dysfunction. Thus, the side effects of morphine, including sedation, may be synergistic with or mask the same symptoms produced by a growing mass lesion in the brain. Furthermore, narcotic agents by decreasing respirations and increasing PCO_2 increase intracranial pressure and may exacerbate the symptoms of brain tumours. Nevertheless, pain in patients with neurological complications of cancers must be treated and must be treated vigorously.

In general, pain in patients suffering neurological symptoms may be divided into two broad categories, systemic pain and neuropathic pain [108]. The importance of distinguishing between the two is that the former responds better to opiates, the latter to drugs such as the tricyclic antidepressants. For systemic pain, one should begin with a mild, peripherally acting analgesic such as acetaminophen, aspirin or the non-steroidal anti-inflammatories. It is probably unwise to use the latter two in patients on glucocorticoids because there may be synergistic actions on the gastrointestinal tract. Most cancer pain will not respond to these drugs and one should move quickly to the narcotic agents, beginning with codeine or oxycodone (in conjunction with acetaminophen or aspirin) and, if ineffective, escalating promptly to morphine or morphine-like agents. Large doses of narcotic drugs are sometimes required to control pain and, if they can be given without substantial side effects, they should be used. However, if the pain is relieved by other means (e.g., direct attack on the tumour), the same dose of narcotic that was previously tolerated may produce excessive sedation and even respiratory insufficiency. Also, if the pain is relieved by other means, the patient may cease taking his narcotics abruptly and, if tolerant, may suffer withdrawal unless the physician instructs the patient to taper the drugs even in the absence of pain.

Neuropathic pain (e.g., that produced by invasion of nerves by tumour - brachial plexopathy for example) is often exceedingly difficult to treat and responds poorly to most narcotic agents. Tricyclic antidepressants, sometimes at surprisingly low doses (e.g., 10 to 25 mg at bedtime), may be more effective than

the narcotic agents. Sometimes a combination of the two is required. The effect of tricyclic antidepressant agents on neuropathic pain appears to be independent of its effect on mood.
Corticosteroids have been advocated for the treatment of bone pain and pain of nerve compression as well. In one controlled trial, corticosteroids produced a significant reduction in both pain and analgesic consumption when compared with a placebo. The response to high-dose intravenous corticosteroids in patients with epidural spinal cord compression is particularly dramatic.

Psychotropic Drugs

Anxiety and depression are significant complications of cancer and, in particular, of its neurological complications [109-111]. Many physicians are reluctant to treat psychological distress, particularly depression, in patients with cancer in the false belief that anxiety or depression, which the physician believes is appropriate for the patient's situation, do not respond to drug therapy. In fact, antidepressant drugs are quite effective in treating depression associated with cancer and anxiolytic drugs also appear to be effective in treating anxiety [110]. Many patients are both anxious and depressed and suffer insomnia as well as anorexia. Tricyclic antidepressants with sedative properties, such as amitriptyline, are often extremely effective in such patients. Given as a single dose at night and gradually increasing from 25 mg to 100 mg, the patient receives both the sedative and the antidepressant effects of the drug. The sedative effects work immediately and patients often feel substantially better after their first good night's sleep. Antidepressant effects take somewhat longer but are still effective. The role of newer anxiolytic antidepressant agents, such as alprazolam and fluoxetine, remain to be elucidated. At low dose most of these drugs appear to have minimal side effects in this particular population.

Constipation

Laxatives are particularly important in neurological complications of cancer, particularly in patients on glucocorticoids. In addition to the general distress produced by constipation, there is substantial evidence that perforation of the bowel (usually sigmoid colon) occurs in constipated patients being treated with steroids for spinal cord compression. Strong efforts should be made to maintain bowel function in patients who are on corticosteroids. In some patients in whom opioids have produced severe constipation, oral naloxone [112,113] appears to relieve constipation without altering the analgesic effect of the corticosteroids. Virtually all patients on opioids, and those who are not but who are constipated, should be on a stool softener and laxatives should be administered ad lib to maintain normal bowel function. Patients should be encouraged to increase bulk in their diet and to take adequate liquids to maintain softening of the stool.

Taste

A number of studies have implicated disordered taste function as a cause of anorexia in patients with cancer and, in particular, in patients undergoing chemotherapy. DeWys and Walters [114] found that one-half of 50 patients with cancer reported a subjective decline in taste sensitivity and 17 were shown to have an increased sweet threshold and reduced bitter threshold. A more recent study, however, in 12 patients with untreated cancer of the oesophagus with 14 matched controls, showed no difference in taste threshold [115]. Abnormal taste may be associated with chemotherapy [116] and may sometimes lead to vomiting. Conditioned taste aversion along with anticipatory nausea and vomiting represent significant problems in patients receiving chemotherapy.

REFERENCES

1 Bruera E, Roca E, Cedaro L, Carraro S, Chacon R: Action of oral methylprednisolone in terminal cancer patients: A prospective randomized double-blind study. Cancer Treat Rep 1985 (69):751-754

2 Della Cuna GR, Pellegrini A, Piazzi M: Effect of methylprednisolone sodium succinate on quality of life in preterminal cancer patients: A placebo-controlled, multicenter study. Exp J Cancer Clin Oncol 1989 (25):1817-1821

3 Tannock I, Gospodarowicz M, Meakin W, Panzarella T, Stewart L, Rider W: Treatment of metastatic prostatic cancer with low-dose prednisone: Evaluation of pain and quality of life as pragmatic indices of response. J Clin Oncol 1989 (7):590-597

4 Popiela T, Lucchi R, Giongo F: Methylprednisolone as palliative therapy for female terminal cancer patients. Exp J Cancer Clin Oncol 1989 (25):1823-1829

5 Cassileth PA, Lusk EJ, Torri S, DiNubile N, Gerson SL: Antiemetic efficacy of dexamethasone therapy in patients receiving cancer chemotherapy. Arch Int Med 1983 (143):1347-1349

6 Markman MD, Scheidler V, Ettinger DS, Quaskey SA, Mellits ED: Antiemetic efficacy of dexamethasone. N Engl J Med 1984 (311):549-552

7 Kardinal CG, Loprinzi CL, Schaid DJ, Hass AC, Dose AM, Athmann LM, Mailliard JA, McCormack GW, Gerstner JB, Schray MF: A controlled trial of cyprohepatidine in cancer patients with anorexia and/or cachexia. Cancer 1990 (65):2657-2662

8 Elrington GM, Murray NMF, Spiro SG, Newsom-Davis J: Neurological paraneoplastic syndromes in patients with small cell lung cancer. A prospective survey of 150 patients. J Neurol Neurosurg Psychiat 1991 (54):764-767

9 Bruera E, Brennis C, Michaud M, Rafter J, Magnan A, Tennant A, Hanson J, Macdonald RN: Association between asthenia and nutritional status, lean body mass, anemia, psychological status, and tumor mass in patients with advanced breast cancer. J Pain Sympt Manag 1989 (4):59-63

10 Bruera E, MacDonald RN: Asthenia in patients with advanced cancer. J Pain Sympt Manag 1988 (3):9-14

11 Lowry SF, Moldawer LL: Tumor necrosis factor and other cytokines in the pathogenesis of cancer cachexia. Prin Prac Oncology 1990 (4):1-12

12 Balis FM, Lester CM, Chrousos GP, Heideman RL, Poplack DG: Differences in cerebrospinal fluid penetration of corticosteroids: possible relationship to the prevention of meningeal leukemia. J Clin Oncol 1987 (5):202-207

13 Jacobs TP, Whitlock RT, Edsall J, Holub DA: Addisonian crisis while taking high-dose glucocorticoids. JAMA 1988 (260):2082-2109

14 Peters WP, Holland JF, Senn H, Rhomberg W, Banerjee L: Corticosteroid administration and localized leukocyte mobilization in man. New Engl J Med 1972 (282):342-345

15 Lane RJM, Mastaglia FL: Drug-induced myopathies in man. The Lancet 1978 (ii):562-565

16 Chalk JB, Ridgeway K, Brophy TRO'O, Yelland JDN, Eadie MJ: Phenytoin impairs the bioavailability of dexamethasone in neurological and neurosurgical patients. J Neurol Neurosurg Psychiat 1984 (47):1087- 1090

17 Lawson LA, Blouin RA, Smith RB, Rappa RP, Young AB: Phenytoin- dexamethasone interaction: a previously unreported observation. Surg Neurol 1981 (16):23-24

18 Brooks SM, Werk EE, Ackerman SJ, Sullivan I, Thrasher K: Adverse effects of phenobarbital on corticosteroid metabolism in patients with bronchial asthma. New Engl J Med 1972 (286):1125-1128

19 Axelrod L: Glucocorticoid therapy. Medicine 1976 (55):39-65

20 Marshall LF, King J, Langfitt TW: The complications of high-dose corticosteroid therapy in neurosurgical patients: A prospective study. Ann Neurol 1977 (1):201-203

21 Oikarinen AI, Uitto J, Oikarinen J: Glucocorticoid action on connective tissue: from molecular mechanisms to clinical practice. Medical Biol 1986 (64):221-230

22 Taylor LP, Posner JB: Steroid myopathy in cancer patients treated with dexamethasone. Neurology 1989 (39 Suppl 1):129

23 Bowyer SL, LaMothe MP, Hollister JR: Steroid myopathy: Incidence and detection in a population with asthma. J Allergy Clin Med 1985 (76):234-242

24 Horber FF, Scheidegger JR, Grunig BE, Frey FJ: Thigh muscle mass and function in patients treated with glucocorticoids. Eur J Clin Invest 1985 (15):302-307

25 Khaleeli AA, Edwards RHT, Gohil K, McPhail G, Rennie MJ, Round J, Ross EJ: Corticosteroid myopathy: a clinical and pathological study. Clin Endocrin 1983 (18):155-166

26 Asaki A, Vignos PJ, Moskowitz RW: Steroid myopathy in connective tissue disease. Am J Med 1976 (61):485-492

27 Coomes EN: The rate of recovery of reversible myopathies and the effects of anabolic agents in steroid myopathy. Neurology 1965 (15):523-530

28 Sakai Y, Kobayashi K, Iwata N: Effects of an anabolic steroid and vitamin B complex upon myopathy induced by corticosteroids. Eur J Pharmacol 1978 (52):353-359

29 Stiefel FC, Breitbart WS, Holland JC: Corticosteroids in cancer: Neuropsychiatric complications. Cancer Invest 1989 7(5):479-491

30 Boston Collaborative Drug Surveillance Program: Acute adverse reactions to prednisone in relation to dosage. Clin Pharmacol Ther 1972 (13):694

31 Wolkowitz OM, Rubinow DR, Breier A, et al: Steroid effects in normals: a prospective study. In: Proceedings of the American Psychiatric Association, 139th Meeting, 1986 p 97

32 Lewis DA, Smith RE: Steroid-induced psychiatric syndrome: a report of 14 cases and review of the literature. J Affective Disord 1983 (5):319

33 Varney NR, Alexander B, MacIndoe JH: Reversible steroid dementia in patients without steroid psychosis. Am J Psychiat 1984 (141):369

34 Viswanathan R, Glickman L: Clonazepam in the treatment of steroid-induced mania in a patient

after renal transplantation. New Engl J Med 1989 (320):319-320
35 Pies R: Persistent bipolar illness after steroid administration. Arch Int Med 1981 (141):1987
36 Sharfstein SS, Sack DS, Fauci AS: Relationship between alternate-day corticosteroid therapy and behavioral abnormalities. JAMA 1982 (248):2987
37 Falk WE, Mahnke MW, Poskanger DC: Lithium prophylaxis of corticotropin-induced psychosis. JAMA 1979 (241):1011
38 Lukert BP, Raisz LG: Glucocorticoid-induced osteoporosis: Pathogenesis and management. Ann Int Med 1990 (22):352-364
39 Engel IA, Straus DJ, Lacher M, et al: Osteonecrosis in patients with malignant lymphoma. A review of 25 cases. Cancer 1981 (48):1245
40 Fast A, Alon M, Weiss S, Zer-Aviv FR: Avascular necrosis of bone following short-term dexamethasone therapy for brain edema. J Neurosurg 1984 (61):983
41 Pocock NA, Eisman JA, Dunstan CR, et al: Recovery from steroid-induced osteoporosis. Ann Int Med 1987 (107):319
42 Felsen DT, Anderson JJ: A cross-study evaluation of association between steroid dose and bolus steroids and avascular necrosis of bone. The Lancet 1987 (i):902-905
43 Reid IR, Alexander CJ, King AR, Ibbertson HK: Prevention of steroid-induced osteoporosis with (3-amino-1-hydroxypropylidene)-1, 1-bisphosphonate (APD). The Lancet 1988 (i):143-146
44 Kaneda A, Yamaura I, Kamikozuru M, Nakai O: Paraplegia as a complication of corticosteroid therapy. J Bone Joint Surg 1984 (66- A):783-785
45 Russell NA, Belanger G, Benoit BG, Latter DN, Finestone DL, Armstrong GW: Spinal epidural lipomatosis: A complication of glucocorticoid therapy. Can J Neurol Sci 1984 (11):383-386
46 Bluming AZ, Zeegen PL: Cataracts induced by intermittent Decadron used as an antiemetic. J Clin Oncol 1986 (4):221-223
47 Shlansky HH, Kolvert G, Gartner S: Exophthalmos induced by steroids. Arch Ophthal 1967 (77):579-581
48 Newsome DA, Eong VG, Cameron TP: "Steroid-induced" mydriasis and ptosis. Invest Ophthal 1971 (10):424-429
49 Akingbehin AO: Corticosteroid-induced ocular hypertension. II. An acquired form. Br J Ophthalmol 1982 (66):541-545
50 Messer J, Reitman D, Sacks HS, et al: Association of adrenocorticosteroid therapy and peptic-ulcer disease. N Engl J Med 1983 (309):21
51 Sauer EG, Dearing WH, Wollaeger EE: Serious untoward gastrointestinal manifestations possibly related to administration of cortisone and corticotropin. Proc Staff Meet Mayo Clin 1953 (28):641
52 Dodi G, Farini R, Pedrazzoli S, Annini G, Naccarato R, Lise M, Fagiolo U: Effect of cimetidine on steroid experimental peptic ulcers. Acta Hepato-Gastroenterol 1978 (25):395-397
53 Camarri E, Chirone E, Benvenuti C: Double-blind placebo controlled cross-over study on cimetidine-prophylactic effect in patients under steroid treatment. Int J Clin Pharm Ther Toxicol 1980 (18):258-260
54 Epstein N, Hood DC, Ransohoff J: Gastrointestinal bleeding in patients with spinal cord trauma. J Neurosurg 1981 (54):16-20
55 Tryba M: Side effects of stress bleeding prophylaxis. Am J Med 1989 (86):85-93
56 Vick NA: Letter to the editor. J Neuro-Oncol 1988 (6):199
57 ReMine SG, McIlrath DC: Bowel perforation in steroid-treated patients. Ann Surg 1980 (192):581-586
58 Fadul CE, Lemann W, Thaler HT, Posner JB: Perforation of the gastrointestinal tract in patients receiving steroids for neurological disease. Neurology 1988 (38):348
59 Baethge BA, Lidsky MD: Intractable hiccups associated with high-dose intravenous methylprednisolone therapy. Ann Int Med 1986 (104):58-59
60 LeWitt PA, Barton NW, Posner JB: Hiccup with dexamethasone therapy. Ann Neurol 1982 (12):405-406
61 Comaish S: A case of hypersensitivity to corticosteroids. Br J Derm 1969 (81):919-925
62 Freedman DM, Schocket AL, Chapel N, Gerber JG: Anaphylaxis after intravenous methylprednisolone administration. JAMA 1981 (245):607-608
63 Flavin DK, Frederickson PA, Richardson JW, Merritt TC: Corticosteroid abuse - an unusual manifestation of drug dependence. Mayo Clin Proc 1983 (58):764-766
64 Czerwinski AW, Czerwinski AB, Whitsett TL, Clark ML: Effects of a single, large, intravenous injection of dexamethasone. Clin Pharmacol Ther 1972 (13):638-642
65 Baharav E, Harpaz D, Mittelman M, Lewinski RH: Dexamethasone-induced perineal irritation. New Engl J Med 1986 (314):515
66 Nelson DA: Dangers from methylprednisolone acetate therapy by intraspinal injection. Arch Neurol 1988 (45):804-806
67 Bernat JL, Sadowsky CH, Vincent FM, Nordgren RE, Margolis G: Sclerosing spinal pachymeningitis. J Neurol Neurosurg Psychiat 1976 (39):1124-1128
68 Henkin RI: Effects of ACTH, adrenocorticosteroids and thyroid hormone on sensory function. In: Stumpf WE, Grant LD (eds) Anatomical Neuroendocrinology. S Karger, Basel 1975 pp 298-316
69 Amatruda TT, Hurst MH, D'Esopo ND: Certain endocrine and metabolic facets of the steroid withdrawal syndrome. J Clin Endocr 1965 (25):1207-1217
70 Dixon RA, Christy NP: On the various forms of corticosteroid withdrawal syndrome. Am J Med 1980 (68):224-230
71 Rotstein J, Good RA: Steroid pseudorheumatism. Arch Int Med 1957 (99):545-555
72 Walker AE, Adamkiewitcz JJ: Pseudotumor cerebri associated with prolonged corticosteroid therapy: reports of four cases. JAMA 1964 (188):779
73 Johnston I, Gilday DL, Hendrick EB: Experimental effects of steroids and steroid withdrawal on

cerebrospinal fluid absorption. J Neurosurg 1975 (42):690-695
74 Henson JW, Jalaj JK, Walker RW, Stover DE, Fels AOS: Pneumocystis carinii pneumonia in patients with primary brain tumors. Arch Neurol 1991 (48):406-409
75 Graham BS, Tucker WS: Opportunistic infections in endogenous Cushing's syndrome. Ann Int Med 1984 (101):334-338
76 Turnbull DM, Rawlins MD, Weightman D, Chadwick DW: "Therapeutic" serum concentration of phenytoin: the influence of seizure type. J Neurol Neursurg Psychiat 1984 (47):231-234
77 Cohen N, Strauss G, Lew R, Silver D, Recht L: Should prophylactic anticonvulsants be administered to patients with newly-diagnosed cerebral metastases? A retrospective analysis. J Clin Oncol 1988 (6):1621-1624
78 Boarini DJ, Beck DW, VanGilder JC: Postoperative prophylactic anticonvulsant therapy in cerebral gliomas. Neurosurgery 1985 (16):290-292
79 Bollini P, Riva R, Albani F, Ida N, Cacciari L, Bollini C, Baruzzi A: Decreased phenytoin level during antineoplastic therapy: a case report. Epilepsia 1983 (24):75-76
80 Dofferhoff ASM, Berendsen HH, Naalt JVD, Haaxma-Reiche H, Smit EF, Postmus PE: Decreased phenytoin level after carboplatin treatment. Am J Med 1990 (89):247-248
81 Grossman SA, Sheidler VR, Gilbert MR: Decreased phenytoin levels in patients receiving chemotherapy. Am J Med 1989 (87):505-510
82 Warren RD, Bender RA: Drug interactions with antineoplastic agents. Cancer Treat Rep 1977 (61):1231-1241
83 Stilman N, Masdeu JC: Incidence of seizures with phenytoin toxicity. Neurology 1985 (35):1769-1772
84 Pagani JJ, Hayman LA, Bigelow RH, Libshitz HI, Lepke RA, Wallace S: Diazepam prophylaxis of contrast media-induced seizures during computed tomography of patients with brain metastases. AJNR 1983 (4):67-72
85 Schmidt D, Einicke I, Haenel F: The influence of seizure type on the efficacy of plasma concentrations of phenytoin, phenobarbital, and carbamazepine. Arch Neurol 1986 (43):263-265
86 Mattson RH, Cramer JA, Collins JF, Smith DB, Delgado-Escueta AV, Browne TR, Williamson PD, Treiman DM, McNamara JO, McCutchen CB, Homan RW, Crill WE, Lubozynski MF, Rosenthal NP, Mayersdorf A: Comparison of carbamazepine, phenobarbital, phenytoin, and primidone in partial and secondarily generalized tonic-clonic seizures. N Engl J Med 1985 (313):145-151
87 Duncan JS, Shorvon SD, Trimble MR: Effects of removal of phenytoin, carbamazepine, and valproate on cognitive function. Epilepsia 1990 31(5):584-591
88 Zaret BS, Cohen RA: Reversible valproic acid-induced dementia: a case report. Epilepsia 1986 27(3):234-240
89 Delattre J-Y, Safai B, Posner JB: Erythema multiforme and Stevens-Johnson syndrome in patients receiving cranial irradiation and phenytoin. Neurology 1988 (38):194-198
90 Gaffey CM, Chun B, Harvey JC, Manz HJ: Phenytoin-induced systemic granulomatous vasculitis. Arch Pathol Lab Med 1986 (110):131-135
91 Anticonvulsant osteomalacia (editorial).The Lancet 1972 (i):805-806
92 Aldenhovel HG: The influence of long-term anticonvulsant therapy with diphenylhydantoin and carbamazepine on serum gamma-glutamyltransferase, aspartate aminotransferase, alanine aminotransferase and alkaline phosphatase. Eur Arch Psychiatr Neurol Sci 1988 (237):312-316
93 Ahmad S, Laidlaw J, Houghton GW, Richens A: Involuntary movements caused by phenytoin intoxication in epileptic patients. J Neurol Neurosurg Psychiat 1975 (38):225-231
94 Taylor LP, Posner JB: Phenobarbital rheumatism in patients with brain tumor. Ann Neurol 1989 (25):92-94
95 Sachellares JC, Lee SI, Dreifuss FE: Stupor following administration of valproic acid to patients receiving other antiepileptic drugs. Epilepsia 1979 (20):697-703
96 Graus F, Rogers LR, Posner JB: Cerebrovascular complications in patients with cancer. Medicine 1985 (64):16-35
97 Powers SK, Edwards MSB: Prophylaxis of thromboembolism in the neurosurgical patient: a review. Neurosurgery 1982 (10):509-513
98 Ruff RL, Posner JB: The incidence of systemic venous thrombosis and the risk of anticoagulation in patients with malignant gliomas. Trans Amer Neurol Assoc 1982 (106):1-3
99 Swann KW, Black McLP: Deep vein thrombosis and pulmonary emboli in neurosurgical patients: a review. J Neurosurg 1984 (61):1055-106
100 Black McLP, Crowell RM, Abbott WM: External pneumatic calf compression reduces deep venous thrombosis in patients with ruptured intracranial aneurysms. Neurosurgery 1986 (18):25-28
101 Kakkar VV, Corrigan TP, Fossard DP, Sutherland I, Thirwell J: Prevention of fatal postoperative pulmonary embolism by low doses of heparin. The Lancet 1977 (i):567-569
102 Green D, Lee MY, Lim AC, Chmiel JS, Vetter M, Pang T, Chen D, Fenton L, Yarkony GM, Meyer PR Jr: Prevention of thromboembolism after spinal cord injury using low-molecular-weight heparin. Ann Int Med 1990 (113):571-574
103 Swann KW, McL Black P, Baker MF: Management of symptomatic deep venous thrombosis and pulmonary embolism on a neurosurgical service. J Neurosurg 1986 (64):563-567
104 Olin JW, Young J, Graor RA, Ruschhaupt WF, Beven EG, Bay JW: Treatment of deep vein thrombosis and pulmonary emboli in patients with primary and metastatic brain tumors. Arch Int Med 1987 (147):2177-2179
105 Atkinson JLD, Sundt TM, Kazmier FJ, Bowie EJW, Whisnant JP: Heparin-induced thrombocytopenia and thrombosis in ischemic stroke. Mayo Clin Proc 1988 (63):353-361

106 McGehee WG, Klotz TA, Epstein DJ, Rapaport SI: Coumadin necrosis associated with hereditary protein C deficiency. Ann Int Med 1984 (100):59-60

107 Walsh DB, Downing S, Nauta R, Gomes MN: Metastatic cancer. A relative contraindication to vena cava filter placement. Cancer 1987 (59):161-163

108 Cancer pain. In: Payne R, Foley KM (eds) The Medical Clinics of North America, Vol 71. WB Saunders Co, Philadelphia 1987

109 Holland JC, Morrow GR, Schmale A, Derogatis L, Stefanek M, Berenson S, Carpente PF, Breitbart W, Feldstein M: A randomized clinical trial of alprazolam versus progressive muscle relaxation in cancer patients with anxiety and depressive symptoms. J Clin Oncol 1991 (9):1004-1011

110 Carey MP, Burish TG: Etiology and treatment of the psychological side effects associated with cancer chemotherapy: a critical review and discussion. Psychol Bull 1988 (104):307-325

111 Holland JC, Rowland JH (eds) Handbook of Psycho-Oncology. OUP, Oxford 1989

112 Sykes NP: Oral naloxone in opioid-associated constipation. The Lancet 1991 (i):1475

113 Culpepper-Morgan JA, Inturrisi CE, Portenoy RK, Kreek MJ: Oral naloxone treatment of narcotic induced constipation. In: Harris LS (ed) Problems of Drug Dependence 1989. Proceedings of the 51st Annual Scientific Meeting of the Committee on Problems of Drug Dependence. DHHS Publication No 90-1663. NIDA Research Monograph Series, Rockville MD 1990 pp 399-400

114 DeWys WD, Walters K: Abnormalities of taste sensation in cancer patients. Cancer 1975 (36):1888-1896

115 Kamath S, Booth P, Lad TE, Kohrs MB, McGuire WP: Taste thresholds of patients with cancer of the esophagus. Cancer 1983 (52):386-389

116 Fetting JH, Wilcox PM, Sheidler VR, Enterline JP, Donehower RC, Grochow LB: Tastes associated with parenteral chemotherapy for breast cancer. Cancer Treat Rep 1985 (69):1249-1251

Subject Index

FSC
www.fsc.org
MIX
Papier aus verantwortungsvollen Quellen
Paper from responsible sources
FSC® C105338

If you have any concerns about our products,
you can contact us on
ProductSafety@springernature.com

In case Publisher is established outside the EU,
the EU authorized representative is:
Springer Nature Customer Service Center GmbH
Europaplatz 3, 69115 Heidelberg, Germany

Printed by Libri Plureos GmbH
in Hamburg, Germany